THE YOGA BOOK

The
YOGA BOOK

A PRACTICAL GUIDE TO SELF-REALIZATION

STEPHEN STURGESS

Foreword by Swami Kriyananda

MOTILAL BANARSIDASS PUBLISHERS
PRIVATE LIMITED • DELHI

Reprint: Delhi, 2007
First Indian Edition: Delhi, 2004
(First Published in 2002 by Watkins Publishing, UK)

© 2000 WATKINS PUBLISHING LIMITED, LONDON

(Stephen Sturgess has asserted his right under the Copyright, Designs and Patents Act, 1988, to be identified as author of this work.)

All Rights Reserved. No part of this book may be reproduced or utilized in any form or by any means, electronic or mechanical, without prior permission in writing from the Publishers.

ISBN: 978-81-208-1990-0

MOTILAL BANARSIDASS
41 U.A. Bungalow Road, Jawahar Nagar, Delhi 110 007
8 Mahalaxmi Chamber, 22 Bhulabhai Desai Road, Mumbai 400 026
236, 9th Main III Block, Jayanagar, Bangalore 560 011
203 Royapettah High Road, Mylapore, Chennai 600 004
Sanas Plaza, 1302 Baji Rao Road, Pune 411 002
8 Camac Street, Kolkata 700 017
Ashok Rajpath, Patna 800 004
Chowk, Varanasi 221 001

Printed in India
BY JAINENDRA PRAKASH JAIN AT SHRI JAINENDRA PRESS,
A-45 NARAINA, PHASE-I, NEW DELHI 110 028
AND PUBLISHED BY NARENDRA PRAKASH JAIN FOR
MOTILAL BANARSIDASS PUBLISHERS PRIVATE LIMITED,
BUNGALOW ROAD, DELHI 110 007

Contents

Acknowledgements	ix
Dedication	xi
Preface	xii
What Is Yoga? *Foreword by Sri Kriyananda*	xv

1	**The Subtle Bodies and the Chakras**	1
	The Physical Body	1
	The Astral Body	3
	The Causal Body	5
	The Soul	5
	The Chakras: Your Inner Universe	8
	Locating the Chakras	20
2	*Yama*	23
	Ashtanga Yoga: The Eight Limbs of Yoga	23
	The Relationship between *Yama* and *Niyama*	24
	The Principles and Practice of *Yama*	25
	Ahimsa: Non-violence, Non-injury, Non-harming	26
	Satya: Non-lying, Truthfulness	30
	Asteya: Non-stealing	32
	Brahmacharya: Non-sensuality	35
	Aparigraha: Non-attachment, Non-greed	46

3	*Niyama*	50
	Saucha: Cleanliness, Purity	50
	Santosha: Contentment	57
	Tapas: Austerity	62
	Svadhaya: Self-study	66
	Isvarapranidhana: Surrender to God	89
4	*Asana*	110
	What is Hatha Yoga?	111
	Purification	115
	Fasting for Purification	146
	The Yogic Diet	152
	Bandhas	154
	Mudras	158
5	*Pranayama*	169
	Prana, the Vital Energy of the Universe	171
	The Five Life–Forces of the Body	176
	Guidelines for the Practice of *Pranayama*	177
	Swara Yoga	184
	Four Different Methods of Breathing	194
	Hand *Mudras* for controlling the breath	200
	Pranayama Techniques	202
	Pranic Healing	216
6	*Pratyahara*	218
	The Senses	219
	The Practice of *Pratyahara*	223
7	*Dharana*	228
	Achieving *Dharana*	229
	Interiorizing and Concentrating the Mind	233
	Other Techniques that Help Concentration	236

8	*Dhyana*	239
	Why We Need to Meditate	239
	The Practice of Meditation	242
	Kriya Yoga: An Advanced Spiritual Accelerator	262
9	*Samadhi*	269
	The Difference Between Meditation (*Dhyana*) and *Samadhi*	269
	The Stages of *Samadhi*	270
	Further Reading	274
	Useful Addresses	276
	Other Resources	280
	Glossary	282
	Index	293

LIST OF ILLUSTRATIONS

Figure 1	The subtle bodies and the chakras	2
Figure 2	The five sheaths of consciousness	2
Figure 3	Body regions of the five *vayus* (vital airs)	4
Figure 4	The seven chakras (centres of consciousness) are situated in the astral body. Here they are shown in relation to the physical body.	9
Figure 5	The chakras and *nadis* (subtle nerve pathways) in the astral body	11
Figure 6	The endocrine glands	19
Figure 7	The nerve plexuses	21
Figure 8	*Padangushthasana* (toe-balance pose)	41
Figure 9	*Viryastambhanasana* (semen-retention pose)	42
Figure 10	*Bhadrasana* (nobility pose)	44
Figure 11	Chanting with *mala* beads	87
Figure 12	The digestive system, showing the flow of warm salt water in the practice of *shankhaprakshalana*	125
Figure 13	Shankaprakshalana	127
Figure 14	*Pavanamuktasana* (gas- and wind-eliminating pose)	130
Figure 15	*Nauli kriya*	140
Figure 16	*Nabho mudra*	166
Figure 17	*Kechari mudra*	166
Figure 18	*Ustrasana* (camel pose)	180
Figure 19	Yogic breathing	198
Figure 20	Position for meditation seated on a chair	246
Figure 21	*Sukhasana*	247
Figure 22	*Swastikasana*	248
Figure 23	*Siddhasana*	249
Figure 24	*Padmasana* (lotus pose)	251
Figure 25	*Ardha padmasana*	252

Acknowledgements

This book took nearly four years to write. The knowledge and experience I gained from various yogic paths and spiritual disciplines over 23 years inspired me to write a comprehensive book on Ashtanga Yoga to inspire others to raise their consciousness to a higher level so that they will know the purpose of this life and feel God's presence in their hearts.

I give my deepest thanks and appreciation to Jeanne Cook, who spent many hours typing the manuscript for me.

I am profoundly grateful to Sri Kriyananda, who very kindly wrote the Foreword for this book, also for his comments and inspirational support.

I give appreciation and thanks also to all other people who may have contributed to the creation of this book, or who inspired me.

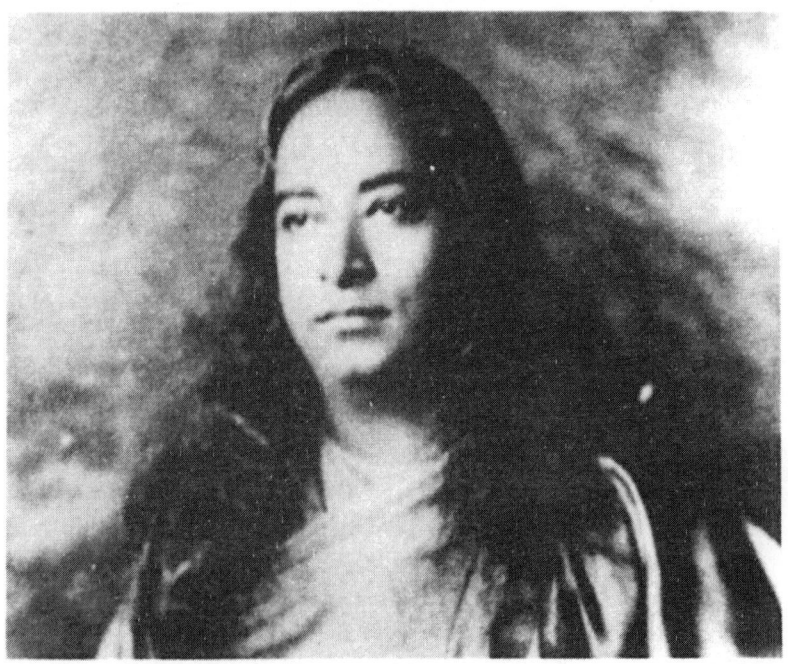

Paramhansa Yogananda

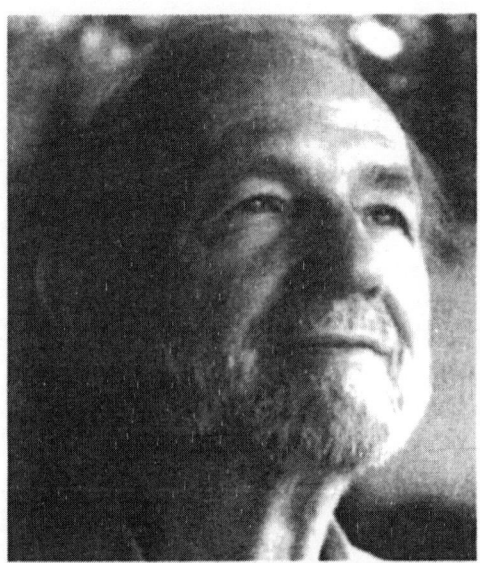

Swami Kriyananda

Dedication

This book is dedicated to my spiritual masters, Jesus Christ, Krishna, Babaji, Lahiri Mahasaya, Swami Sri Yukteswar and my beloved Master Paramhansa Yogananda who has shown me the true path to God.

I also dedicate this book to Sri Kriyananda, who inspired me to follow the Kriya Yoga teachings of Yogananda.

This book is for all my spiritual brothers and sisters at Ananda and for all those who have helped me along the way to Truth.

May this book inspire you, the reader, to live in the consciousness of God, that you may find the true inner joy and inner peace.

Preface

Whether you realize it or not you are a soul, a spiritual being in a physical body. The body is the temple of the soul, and the soul is a reflection of God.

Your true identity, your true nature, is pure consciousness, infinite pure being, which is separate from the physical body, senses or mind-ego; but through ignorance and self-forgetfulness you have imposed limitations and wrong identification upon yourself. Due to ignorance and lifetimes of concentration on the material body, and attraction to the objects of the senses, the Self has forgotten its omnipresent nature.

It is the ego-mind that creates an illusory reality formed by its own thoughts, desires, imagination, memories and ideas, that keeps you from knowing and realizing your true soul-nature, your divinity within. In ignorance, the ego-mind cannot see truth, the divine reality, because it is blinded by its own desires.

It is the false identification of the Self with the body, mind and senses, and your separation from the infinite, that is the cause of all suffering and unhappiness.

Whether knowingly or unknowingly, there are two things in life that everybody wants:

- freedom from pain, suffering and want
- permanent happiness or bliss (joy)

Happiness and joy are the very nature of the Self; the Self is itself the very source of happiness, its nature is pure being – pure consciousness – bliss (*sat–chid–ananda*). There is no happiness in any object of the world. Truth and happiness are not outside you, they are *within* you.

The most important thing to know and do in life is to become consciously aware of your own spiritual, divine nature and your eternal relationship with God, the Father-Mother of creation – to love God with all your heart (feeling), with all your mind (concentration), with all your soul (soul-union through meditation) and with all your strength (attention and energy), and to love your neighbours (all beings, regardless of their colour, beliefs, caste, creed or religion) as yourself.

This book is about Ashtanga Yoga, also known as Raja Yoga, and is not to be confused with the practice which is becoming popular in the West of Ashtanga Vinyasa Asanas, sometimes known as Power Yoga – a dynamic series of connecting movements using *ujjayi* breath and *uddiyana bandha*, made popular by Krishnamacharya and Pattabhi Jois from India. This is a wonderful system to align the skeletal system correctly and to strengthen, revitalize and make the body flexible and to promote health. But if it is practised neglecting the important spiritual aspects of yoga, such as the *yamas* (ethical disciplines) and *niyamas* (moral disciplines) then it reduces yoga to the level of a physical fitness system. This is important to understand because some people are under the misconception that yoga *is* a physical fitness system for achieving outward results – a slim healthy body, sexual energy, magnetism, psychic powers, beauty and longevity. To achieve these outward results only for the purpose of continuing a self-centred sense-oriented life is of no value from a spiritual viewpoint. In the West it seems that the practice of yoga postures (*asanas*) has become synonymous with the totality of yoga. This is an incomplete view and understanding of what true yoga is.

To be understood correctly, yoga postures have to be seen in the context of Patanjali's Eight Limbs of Yoga, that is, as a *spiritual* discipline, which integrates and balances the mind and body. *Asana* means 'posture' and 'seat'. Patanjali's interpretation of the term does not refer to any particular yoga postures, but only to the ability to hold the body motionless and the mind steady, for deep meditation. Hatha Yoga is part of a systematic process towards self-realization, which recognizes that a less than healthy, vitalized body is a distraction, which can obstruct progress towards perfection. In this book, I have included Hatha Yoga practices without going into any detail about yoga postures (*asanas*) because there are many good books on that subject alone.

My spiritual teacher, Sri Kriyananda, has very kindly written an

Introduction for this book, which clearly defines the true aims of yoga. He is a very inspiring spiritual teacher and Kriya yogi (a direct disciple of Paramhansa Yogananda), who has written many inspiring books himself, some of which are listed at the back of this book.

The first chapter of this book begins with the subject of the subtle bodies and the chakras. This is to give you an understanding that there is more to us than our physiology and psychology. From the beginning of the book, you will be drawn in from a spiritual perspective.

The chapters that follow deal with eight 'limbs' of yoga, a scientific and practical system formulated by the ancient illumined sage Patanjali from the ancient oral traditions, which leads the seeker to his or her own Self-realization. It takes you step by step through eight stages of yoga culminating in *samadhi*, in a simple, clear and direct way.

These time-proven teachings give methods and techniques for purifying the mind and body to attain higher states of consciousness, for achieving the goal of Self-realization. Let us always remember to keep in mind the true aim and purpose of yoga – to remove the obstacles, to dispel the ignorance that obscures the true inner Self as knowledge, through the practice of uninterrupted awareness and discrimination between what is real and what is unreal.

We are individualized expressions of God's light, love, peace and wisdom, we are ever-existing, ever-conscious, ever-new bliss. Affirm that you are eternal, ever-pure, full of knowledge, full of strength, full of blessedness.

Remember, your purpose in life is to realize your divinity, to awaken to the God within you. To realize and express that pure consciousness that you truly are, you need to purify the mind and body and resolve to meditate deeply on a regular basis every day to clear the mind of distractions. You must sincerely want to awaken, aspire to the highest truth and expand your consciousness. Yoga is no part-time exercise; once taken up, it involves your entire life. This total approach to life reveals your commitment to awakening in self-realization. If we are unmotivated, uncommitted and practise half-heartedly, we cannot expect complete success and fulfilment in life.

May you awaken to the true path of happiness and joy within you.

Stephen Sturgess (Shankara)
November 1996

Foreword

What is Yoga?
by Sri Kriyananda

Great truths are universally relevant, and consequently defy every narrowing attempt at definition. Take, as the sublime example, love – God Himself – or, at a more prosaic level, such seemingly mechanical functions of Nature as gravity and electromagnetism.

Such a truth – and in fact one closely related to love – is yoga. Yoga, a Sanskrit word, means union. From this root is derived our own English word yoke. The union implied here is an eternal truth. It is not something to be achieved by artifice, such as couples uniting in wedlock or nations uniting on the strength of peace treaties. Indeed, unless such outward unions are based on a recognition of deeper, already existing bonds, they will be short-lived. True union can only be recognized; it cannot be created.

Yoga dignifies the essential unity that is the basis of life. Like love, this great truth embraces the full spectrum of reality, from the most spiritual to the most material. In the highest sense, yoga, as spiritual union, signifies the soul's union with God. At the opposite end of the spectrum it embraces the affinity of atomic particles for one another. Like love, moreover, the deeper reality implied is always spiritual, even when treating of seemingly inanimate matter.

Both love and yoga can be understood better through their active expression then by static definition. They are experiential truths, and not mere abstractions.

The practice of yoga, then, is a process of self-discovery. It is an awakening of long-somnolent memories of who and what we *really* are: within ourselves, an integral whole; externally, an integral part of all that is. The benefit of yoga practice is no mere creation of a new persona.

In this emphasis on self-awareness, as opposed to self-development, yoga stands diametrically opposed to most of the assumptions of our age. For modern thought accepts with Darwin the concept that evolution is progressive in a linear sense; that it is born of struggle, and accompanied by tension, anguish and pain. Progress, on the other hand, conceived of as a voyage of self-discovery, implies a retreat from tension and reduction of suffering, offering instead the deep peace that comes with true self-recognition and acceptance. Thus, the *Bhagavad Gita* states, 'Even a little practice of this religion frees one from dire fears and colossal suffering.'

The spiritual practice or 'religion', here referred to is yoga. As Krishna is quoted as saying, 'Arjuna, be thou a yogi.' True yoga practice is that which is based on attitudes of inner relaxation and calmness.

Yoga, then, rightly understood, is not a practice for achieving outward results: slimness, poise, muscular co-ordination, or the development of artistic or intellectual skills. Such gains, if sought purely for themselves, cannot but be short-lived. They are, however, natural results of the recognition of union as an inner and fundamental truth of life. For they are normal manifestations of a nature that is self-integrated. The difference lies in the focus of one's aspirations. Unlike so many modern schools of self-development, yoga practice does not add such outward benefits strenuously to a growing arsenal of skills and accomplishments. It draws one to a state of rest at one's own centre, from which centredness all that is rightfully one's own is achieved effortlessly.

Yoga, as union, implies perfect harmony of body, mind and spirit. On a physical level, it implies glowing health. On a mental level, it implies the harmonious integration of the personality, and the corresponding elimination of psychological 'complexes'. On the soul level, yoga implies union of the little self with the greater Self, of the ego with the vastness of cosmic awareness, and, as stated earlier, of the individual soul with its infinite Source: God.

The different paths of yoga all have this total union for their goal. They differ only in the matter of emphasis.

Karma Yoga, the path of action, teaches one how to live in a spirit of self-integration, even while engaged in strenuous activity. The teachings of Karma Yoga are valid for everyone, for they deal with an aspect of life that concerns everyone, even the meditative yogi. (For are not thoughts, too, a form of action?)

Gyana Yoga (often written 'Jnana Yoga'), the path of discrimination and wisdom, teaches one how to achieve a sense of inner integration on a mental level. Thought, too, is an activity engaged in by all. The teachings of Gyana Yoga, then, have universal relevance.

Bhakti Yoga, the path of devotion, deals also with a fundamental aspect of human nature: feeling, and the way to refine emotions into pure, self-giving love. Without devotion, indeed, action becomes sterile, and discrimination sinks to the passive level of mere armchair philosophy.

Hatha Yoga, often described as the physical path of yoga, is not really a distinct path at all, but rather the physical branch of the meditative science of Raja Yoga. As such, it must be understood as a means of awakening and freeing the inner energies of the body, that they may be directed toward the higher activity of divine contemplation. Essentially, the goal of *asana* or yoga posture, in Hatha Yoga is simply the ability to sit still with a straight spine, and with the body relaxed. The yoga postures then, are primarily intended to help one to achieve complete physical, and subsequently mental and emotional, relaxation.

Raja Yoga, the path of meditation, is the central teaching of yoga, hence its name: Raja, meaning 'royal'. Perfection in each of the other branches of yoga results, however indirectly, in superconscious awareness. But superconsciousness is the direct aim of Raja Yoga, through techniques of concentration that help to lift one above the identity with body, mind, feelings and ego.

There is a fundamental misunderstanding in the West, particularly among Christians, namely the belief that yoga practice implies a rejection of divine grace. Indeed, it would be absurd to imagine that union with God could be achieved by imposing oneself on the Lord with or without His consent! As a matter of fact, *kripa,* or divine grace, is a concept so fundamental to Hinduism that its omission is more often an attempt to correct a widespread tendency to rely too heavily on grace, at the expense of self-effort.

The Yoga Sutras of Patanjali, the fundamental scripture of yoga, begins with the statement, 'Now we come to the study of yoga.' The implication of that word 'now' is that the study of yoga follows properly upon the recognition and acceptance of other basic life values. To practise yoga successfully, as is well understood in India, one must be already steeped in certain attitudes, among which would be included such presumptively 'Christian' virtues as faith, devotion, humility, and a deep love for the longing to commune with God.

I recommend to all readers of this book, therefore, a yogic approach to it. Look upon this ancient science, in other words, not as a study apart from the life you normally live, but as integral to every aspect of it, even the most familiar and mundane.

1

THE SUBTLE BODIES AND THE CHAKRAS

Although our physical bodies appear to be dense and solid, at the most fundamental level they are composed of trillions of molecules and atoms, or energy in constant transformation. In addition to the physical body, the soul (the in-dwelling pure spirit – the reality of who we really are) has several interdependent non-physical, subtle bodies or vehicles surrounding and interpenetrating the physical form, each of which is a field of energy vibrating at a particular frequency level and density.

The individual soul expresses itself through five sheaths (*koshas*), which are divided between three bodies – the *physical* body and two surrounding subtle bodies, known as the *astral* body and the *causal* body (see figure 1).

The physical, astral and causal bodies serve respectively as mediums for our daily experience in the three states of mind – waking (*jagrat*), dream (*swapna*) and dreamless sleep (*sushupti*). The soul is beyond these three states, being a witness to them.

So there are five sheaths divided between three bodies, which are the vehicles for the expression of the soul consciousness, which is distinct from them all (see figure 2).

THE PHYSICAL BODY

The *annamaya kosha* (the food sheath) is the physical sheath of the gross body, which is subject to birth, growth, disease, decay and death. It is called the food sheath because of its dependence on gross *prana* in the form of food, water and air. (*Prana* is the vital life-energy, which

2 THE YOGA BOOK

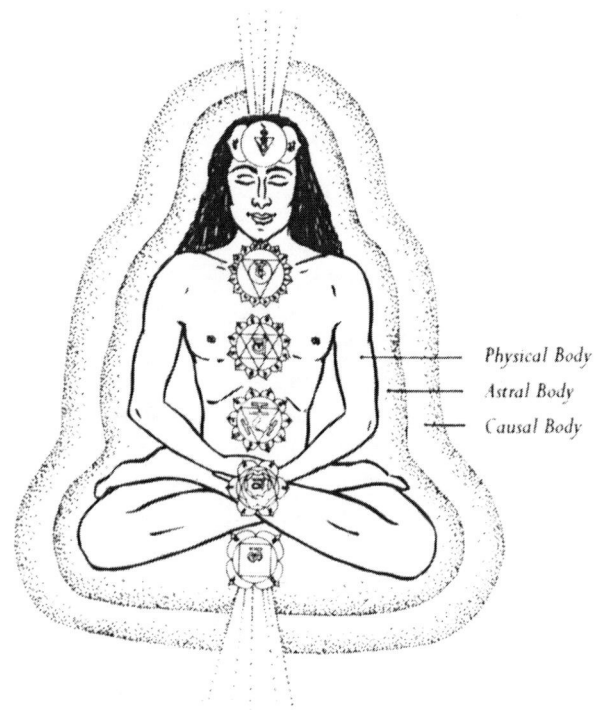

Figure 1 *The subtle bodies and the chakras*

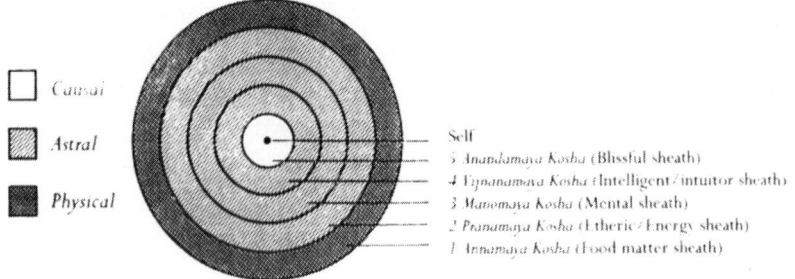

Figure 2 *The five sheaths of consciousness*

sustains life and creation. *Prana* permeates the whole of creation and exists in both the macrocosmos and the microcosmos. Without *prana* there is no life. *Prana* is the link between the astral and physical bodies, when this link is cut off, then death takes place in the physical body. Both the *prana* and the astral body depart from the physical body.) It is also formed by the five elements (ether, air, fire, water and earth).

THE ASTRAL BODY

The astral body is composed of five subtle elements – *akash* (ether), *vayu* (air), *tejas* (fire), *jala* (water) and *prithvi* (earth) – which produce the five gross elements on the physical plane.

The astral body is divided into three sheaths.

THE *PRANAMAYA KOSHA*

This pranic body (the vital or etheric sheath) provides energy and vitalizes the physical body. It is approximately the same size and shape as the physical body.

The vital sheath is composed of five *pranas* (life-energies), which have distinct functions in the working of the physical body (see figure 3).

Vyana, 'outward moving air', is the vital air that regulates the overall movements of the body, co-ordinating the other vital airs. It permeates the whole body.

Udana, 'upward moving air', functions between the throat and the top of the head, activating the organs of sense: eyes, nose, ears, tongue. It has an upward movement that carries the *kundalini shakti* (a person's potential spiritual energy or vital energy force, lying dormant at the base of the spine, in the *muladhara chakra* or base energy centre. This creative, vital energy force passes through the main subtle nerve channel (*sushumna nadi*) in the centre of the spinal cord, when awakened, to the crown chakra (*sahasrara*), the seventh energy centre located at the crown of the head.

At death, *udana* separates the astral body from the physical form.

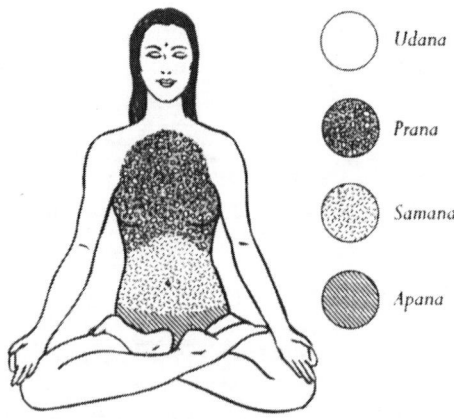

Figure 3 *Body regions of the five vayus (vital airs)*

Prana (vital life-energy) is a specific manifestation of *cosmic prana* (the cosmic life-energy that pervades both the macrocosmic universe and the microcosmic unit of the body). The cosmic prana enters the body through the medulla oblongata at the base of the brain. It then descends and ascends through the astral spine, where it is modified by the chakras and differentiated into the vital airs (*vayus* – pranic air currents).

Prana, 'forward moving air', functions between the throat and the top of the diaphragm, activating the respiration. It also raises the *kundalini shakti* to *udana*.

Samana, 'balancing air', functions in the abdominal area between the navel and the heart, activating and controlling the digestive system, the heart and the circulatory system.

Apana, 'air that moves away', functions from the region of the navel to the feet, activating expulsion and excretion. It has a downward movement, but carries the *kundalini* upwards to unite with *prana*.

These five vital airs (*vayus*) are conjoined with the five subtle organs of action (speech, hands, legs, organs of evacuation and procreation), which have their gross counterparts in the physical body.

THE *MANOMAYA KOSHA*

This is the mental sheath, and is more subtle than the vital pranic sheath. It holds the *annamaya* and *pranamaya koshas* together as an integrated whole. The mental sheath functions as a messenger between each body, communicating the experiences and sensations of the external world to the intelligent sheath, and the influences of the causal and astral bodies to the physical body.

The mental sheath is formed of the volitional mind (*manas*), the subconscious and the five sense organs of perception in their astral form (sight, hearing, smell, taste and touch).

THE *VIJNANAMAYA KOSHA*

The intelligent sheath functions as the knower and the doer, and being the subtlest of all the aspects of the mind, it reflects the radiance of soul consciousness.

It is composed of the cognitive mind (*buddhi*), the intellect and ego conjoined with the five subtle sense organs of perception.

THE CAUSAL BODY

The *anandamaya kosha* (the bliss sheath) is the subtlest and innermost of the three bodies that reflects the blissfulness of the soul. It is the cause of both the subtle and gross bodies.

In dreamless sleep the mind recedes from the physical waking state and the astral dream state to the causal body. It enters a subtle state in profound dreamless sleep, in which the functions of the mind and the sense organs are suspended. In this blissful, restful state there is no sense of ego and no thoughts.

THE SOUL

The soul, in-dwelling self or spirit resides within all three bodies (physical, astral and causal), witnessing all of their activities. The soul is the ever-shining consciousness, perfect and complete, having no limits and without beginning or end.

Death, Samskaras and Karma

At the time of physical death (which is not the end or annihilation of an individual) the soul, or the self, which animates the body, withdraws from the physical form clothed in the astral and causal bodies. The lifeline which transmits life-energy (*prana*) to the physical body becomes severed; the consciousness frees itself from the limitations of the physical and becomes associated with the subtle body.

The soul continues to exist in the vehicle of the astral body (mind, ego, subtle sense organs and vital airs). This carries with it *samskaras* (past impressions) or *karma* of all one's actions, thoughts and desires.

Samskaras are the dormant impressions of our past lives (actions, desires, thoughts and memories) that are linked to the soul with the subconscious mind. Our past *samskaras* motivate our present actions — what we sow, we reap.

Karma comes from the sanskrit root *kri*, meaning 'to do', 'to make', 'to act'. Not only is *karma* the cause and seed for the continuation of the life process after death (rebirth), but even in this present life, our actions or *karma* produce good and bad results, having a decisive influence on our present character and destiny.

The soul is subject to three types of *karma*.

- *sanchita karmas* — those that have accumulated in several previous lifetimes
- *prarabdha karmas* — results of past actions which are producing fruit in the present
- *agami karmas* — the actions which are being done in this present life and will bear fruits in a future life

The *sanchita* and *agami karmas* are destroyed by attaining self-realization (God-realization), but *prarabdha karmas* can only be exhausted by experiencing their fruits in the present life.

Sleep and Death

Every night when we fall asleep, we die to everything we know. Like death, sleep is a transition from the plane of material existence to a plane that is more subtle. What we call death is our impression of

THE SUBTLE BODIES AND THE CHAKRAS

change over which we have no control. Similarly sleep is also a change, but unlike death we gladly surrender, relax and 'let go' into sleep. Why? Because we have done it so many times and remember sleep as being painless and refreshing. But can you remember ever dying?

The awareness of consciousness is continuous, we feel that we existed even during sleep, and when we awaken in the morning we are aware of the 'I' consciousness, which has remained exactly the same as before we went to sleep. The 'I' consciousness or the self has not changed. For a moment or two as we awake from our night's sleep, we may feel disorientated, especially if we have had a very unconscious type of sleep. Then we become more orientated and aware of our familiar surroundings. We awake from the night's dream to begin the day dream, and so it goes on like the cycle of births and deaths.

When we lie down to go to sleep, we are aware of sensations, smell, touch and sounds. Then, as our consciousness begins to withdraw, we fall asleep. The subtle body withdraws from the physical form and the mind-ego and thoughts go into a subtle state. During sleep there is no awareness of the physical body and there is no feeling of pain. It is only when the mind and senses are connected with the body that pain arises. The Self, our true spiritual nature, is not touched by pleasure or pain.

In the second chapter of the *Bhagavad Gita*, Lord Krishna reminds us of our immortal and eternal true nature.

> *As we observe in this life the change of a youthful body to an old one, so too after death, the soul adopts another body. Those who have understood the true nature of life are not deluded by these changes.*
>
> 2:13

> *The indwelling Self never takes birth and will never die. It has always existed and shall never cease to be. For it is birthless, eternal, immortal and unchangeable. It is not slain when the body is killed.*
>
> 2:20

> *As a person discards worn-out clothes and acquires new clothes, so also the embodied soul abandons a worn-out body and enters into another one which is new.*
>
> 2:22

The Self is beyond the power of any weapon to injure or of fire to burn it. It neither becomes moistened by water, nor dried by the winds.

2:23

The Self is indivisible and indissoluble and cannot be transformed by fire or air. The soul is everlasting, omnipresent, unwaveringly steady and ever-existent.

2:24

Realize that the soul, the spirit-self, is unmanifested, it is beyond the mind's ability to conceive and cannot be changed. Therefore, knowing this, transcend your unfounded anxieties and grief.

2:25

THE CHAKRAS: YOUR INNER UNIVERSE

Chakra is a Sanskrit word meaning 'wheel' or 'revolving disc'. The *chakras* are subtle revolving vortices of energy, situated within the astral body. They connect the five sheaths (*koshas*) that embody the soul, to the functions of the physical body, primarily through the endocrine glands and the nerve plexuses in the spine.

The chakras serve as transformers and act as regulators to receive, assimilate and distribute energy (pranic life-force) to the subtle body, which then distributes the energy to the spinal nerve plexuses where it is in turn transferred to the blood circulation and organs of the physical body.

The subtle pranic life-force enters the body at the base of the brain (medulla oblongata) and flows to the higher brain centres. Then it filters downward through the six major chakras or energy centres. As this energy and light filters and spirals down through each chakra, it increasingly becomes more dense. At the lowest chakra at the base of the spine (*muladhara chakra*), the vibrational frequency is lower and slower than at those above it. The higher the chakra, the more subtle and finer the vibrational frequency. These higher chakras are closely related to the innermost sheaths and higher levels of consciousness.

The energy that filters down through the chakras, ultimately spirals down from cosmic energy, produced from cosmic light, which is

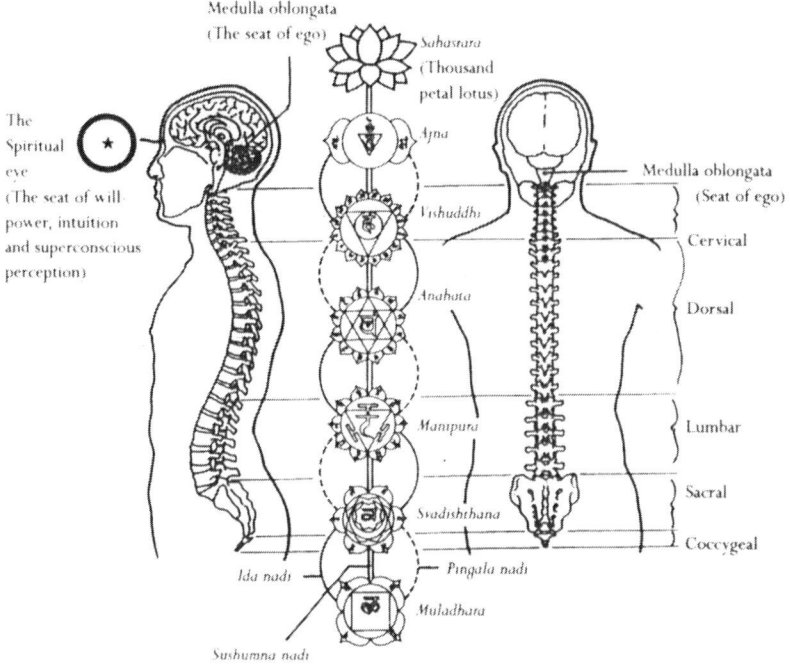

Figure 4 *The seven chakras (centres of consciousness) are situated in the astral body. Here they are shown in relation to the physical body.*

created by the will and energy of God – the Cause of all cause.

Consciousness descends in a spiralling movement of energy and, as it descends, subdivides and stretches out, it becomes matter. Consciousness moving becomes energy and when the movement is slowed down, it becomes matter. As it condenses into matter it forms the five elements: ether (space), air, fire, water and earth – first the subtle elements, then the gross elements. The difference between one element and the other is a difference in their vibratory wavelength frequencies.

As consciousness descends and moves in space, it becomes air. When air moves there is friction and therefore fire, and when the gases collide and fire is generated, water is also generated; and then water condenses into solid substances (earth).

The chakras represent these subtle elements. For their position in relation to the physical body, see figure 4. The earth centre (*muladhara chakra*) is that part of your anatomy which comes into contact with the earth. A little above there is the water element (*swadisthana chakra*), the next subtle element, located where water collects. At the navel centre (*manipura chakra*) is the fire region – when we talk about digestion, we think of the gastric fire there. Above the navel is the heart region (*anahata chakra*), which represents air – the region in which the lungs and oxygenation operate. Above the heart is the throat region (*vishuddhi chakra*) – a little space (ether) in the throat. Higher still is the spiritual eye (*ajna chakra*) at the point between the eyebrows, which represents the mind.

The chakras vibrate at different frequencies as they transmit energy. Each is associated with a vibrational frequency, a characteristic colour, a sound, an element, a planet, a spiritual quality and a presiding deity.

Kundalini Yoga, Laya Yoga, Tantric Yoga and Kriya Yoga are the main branches of yoga that specifically concentrate on the chakras. On the path of Kriya Yoga as taught by Paramhansa Yogananda and his great line of Kriya Masters, the chakras are concentrated on in the higher techniques of Kriya meditation.

There are psychic people and advanced yogis who have the psychic vision to see these subtle energy centres and fields of energy as they look into the auric field of a person. They see the chakras as funnels of dynamic, revolving vortices of energy and light, with colours, moving rapidly in cross-section.

THE *NADIS*

The chakras are connected to the physical body by subtle nerve channels (*nadis*) located in the astral body and invisible to the physical eye. The subtle solar plexus in the astral body is the centre from which 72,000 (350,000 according to the *Shiva Samhita*, 2:13) *nadis*, invisible energy currents, flow out to the entire subtle circuitry of the astral body (see figure 5). The solar plexus is the main storage battery of *prana* and large amounts of *prana* can be stored to give vitality to the body, through the practice of *pranayama*. The *nadis* can be purified by this practice particularly through *anuloma viloma pranayama*

The Subtle Bodies and the Chakras 11

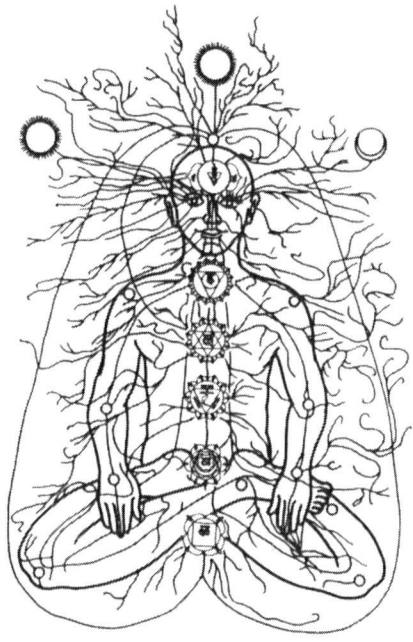

Figure 5 *The chakras and nadis (subtle nerve pathways) in the astral body*

(alternate nostril breathing). If the *nadis* are not purified, then the *prana* cannot flow into the *sushumna nadi*.

The life-energy or *prana* which flows through the *nadis* is used by the soul in its expression through the physical and astral manifestations. Without the light of the in-dwelling self or soul, the brain, mind, body organs and even *prana* cannot function. It is the self that sustains the body by the agency of *prana*.

The three primary *nadis* that connect the chakras together are the *sushumna*, the *ida* and the *pingala*. The *ida* (negative lunar current) begins at the *muladhara chakra* on the left side of the *sushumna*, and the *pingala* (positive solar current), begins at the *muladhara chakra* on the right side of the *sushumna*. They cross each other at the junction of each chakra, like the two snakes of the caduceus, and meet at the *ajna chakra*. The chakras are polarized by the upward and downward movement of energy through the *ida* and *pingala nadis*. Paramhansa Yogananda stated in his *Autobiography of a Yogi* that the six chakras become 12 by polarity, corresponding to the twelve signs of the zodiac.

The Major Chakras

The six important chakras are positioned horizontally within the astral spine (*sushumna nadi*). They are transformers for the main dynamo of energy, the seventh and highest chakra, the *sahasrara chakra* (1,000-petalled lotus), located in the upper brain and beyond. This crown chakra is often illustrated in portraits of saints and Jesus, the Christ, as a halo of bright light around and over the head, indicating illumination and liberation of consciousness.

The chakras are also referred to metaphorically in the yoga scriptures as lotuses, their rays of energy forming the petals. Each chakra has a certain number of petals. In the ordinary person whose mind is operating in the lower centres or planes of consciousness, these petals are turned downwards, their rays of energy flowing out toward the senses.

The yogi, through yoga practice (Asana, Pranayama, Kriya meditation) and right attitude turns the petals upward, pointing toward the brain, creating an upward flow of energy to the higher chakras. Sri Kriyananda says in his *14 Steps to Joy*, 'Right attitude keeps the whirlpool of self-realization expanding outward to infinity, instead of becoming locked in a narrow cycle of ego-limitation.'

The dormant *kundalini* pranic energy stored at the base of the spine is awakened by the practice of yoga techniques, spiritual practices (*sadhana*) with a spiritual consciousness. When this powerful *kundalini* energy is activated it rises upwards through the astral spinal pathway piercing each chakra as it ascends. When the *kundalini* reaches the highest chakra at the crown of the head (*sahasrara*) the yogi becomes perfectly detached from his or her body and mind, and enters into *nirvikalpa samadhi*, the blissful superconscious state in which the yogi realizes his or her oneness with God. In this state the enlightened yogi is freed from all limitations caused by time and space. After the experience of this *samadhi*, the yogi continues to live and move in the world like any other person, but with one difference: the yogi's consciousness is always of the highest realization, in which there is no distinction between him or her and God.

The *Muladhara Chakra* (First Centre)

The *muladhara chakra* is also referred to as the base or root centre. The Sanskrit word *mula* (pronounced 'moola') means root. It is the first chakra located at the base of the spinal column, where the dormant *kundalini* is likened to a serpent which rests in a coil, and like a spring can release its potential energy when it strikes. When *kundalini* is aroused, she awakens, uncoils and begins her journey upwards, piercing each chakra as she ascends, until she merges with *shiva* (consciousness) in divine union (*samadhi*) in the *sahasrara chakra* (crown centre).

Muladhara is symbolized by a deep red lotus with four petals. Inside the lotus is a yellow square and within the square is a downward-pointing triangle.

This chakra embodies the earth element (symbolized by the yellow square) because it is the grossest part of the body, concerned with the physical body and the material plane. It has the qualities of solidity and inertia. It is also the seat of *annamaya kosha*, the sheath of nourishment, connected with the absorption of food and elimination of fecal matter. It is related to the sense of smell.

The *muladhara chakra* is concerned with basic existence and survival instincts: feelings of fear, guilt, paranoia, personal security, food, shelter, defensiveness, aggression, gratification of the senses, the instinctive drive to have sex and reproduce. An example of the most basic survival instincts and energy centred in the *muladhara chakra* is the animal which lives in the wild with its primitive responses to life-threatening situations. It hunts and kills another animal to eat it, or it fears being hunted itself.

It is here, also in this centre, that our lowest *samskaras* (deep mental impressions produced by past experiences) and *karma* (past actions, which will lead to certain results in a cause-and-effect relationship) are embedded.

The *Swadhisthana Chakra* (Second Centre)

The Sanskrit word *swa* means 'one's own' and *adhisthana* means 'dwelling place' so *swadhisthana* means 'one's own abode'.

Swadhisthana is the second chakra, located in the sacral region of the spine, at the level of the coccyx, behind the sexual organs. It is associated with the element of water and physiologically related to the urinary system, sexual organs and reproductive systems.

Swadhisthana is symbolized as a six-petalled vermilion or orange-red lotus, within which is a white crescent moon, symbolizing the element of water and the unconscious mind.

Swadhisthana is the seat of *pranamaya kosha*.

The sense connected with this chakra is taste, which is also related to the sexual organs, because the taste of food stimulates our emotions, which can create exciting, pleasurable sensations. If a person has his or her energy focused in this chakra they will be preoccupied with sensuality and sexuality – they will be seeking sensual pleasure, whether it be food sensations, sexual pleasure or excitement.

The consciousness of feelings primarily experienced in this chakra is both pleasurable and painful – feelings of vulnerability, the longing to feel loved and emotionally secure, fear of being rejected, loneliness, sensual and sexual desires, romantic feelings, emotional insecurity.

The way to rise above sensual and sexual desires is to transmute the sexual energy into more creative and refined spiritual forms of expression. We need to rechannel our passionate self-seeking inwardly into compassion and selfless service so that the heart unfolds, and a higher spiritual love begins to manifest.

The *Manipura Chakra* (Third Centre)

The Sanskrit word *manipura* is derived from two words, *mani* meaning 'jewel' and *pura* meaning 'city'. *Manipura* means 'city of jewels'.

This is the third chakra, located opposite the navel, in the spine. It is related to the solar plexus, which controls the digestive fire and heat regulation in the body. It radiates and distributes pranic energy throughout the entire body systems. It is also the seat of *pranamaya kosha*.

Manipura is symbolized as a ten-petalled bright yellow lotus. In the centre of the lotus is an inverted red triangle that symbolizes the fire element. This chakra is a centre of power, energy, will and achievement. Here we have both the fire of desire and the power of emotions to deal with. Ego-centred consciousness with its arrogance, anger,

The Subtle Bodies and the Chakras 15

power games and desire to control, possess and dominate is the negative quality associated with the third chakra.

As we purify our consciousness and expand our awareness, our emotional life becomes more integrated and channelled towards a more positive and higher consciousness.

Manipura is related to the sense of sight.

The *Anahata Chakra* (Fourth Centre)

The Sanskrit word *anahata* literally means 'unstruck'. It refers to the inner subtle sound vibration (*nada*) experienced in meditation. It is called 'unstruck' because it is not created by physical friction.

There are two kinds of *nada*:
- *ahat nada*, all external or struck sounds, such as musical instruments played
- *anahata nada*, all sounds which do not have any external source, or 'unstruck' sound

The *anahata chakra* is the fourth centre, located at the level of the heart. It is symbolized as a blue lotus with 12 petals. Its element, air, is located in the smoke-coloured centre, within which are two intersecting triangles, representing the higher and lower aspects of our nature. In Judaism, this triangle symbol is called the Star of David.

The *anahata chakra* is known as the heart centre, the centre of spiritual or divine love. When this chakra is fully awakened love is experienced as being unconditional, selfless and compassionate.

Many of the great saints and sages who have fully awakened the heart chakra give great importance to developing the natural love of the heart: to love all beings as expressions of God's omnipresence. By opening our hearts to God's love, we become love.

The great celestial sage Narada wrote in his *Sutras on the Philosophy of Love*:

> *The path of love is the highest path.*
> *Love of God is supreme; devotion to God*
> *is devotion to eternal truth.*

Sutra 81

Yogananda's guru, Swami Sri Yukteswar said:

> Until one develops the natural love of the heart, it is impossible to take a single step on the spiritual path.

Jesus Christ said:

> Love the Lord thy God with all thy heart and with all thy soul, and with all thy mind.

The heart chakra is a point of transition between the three lower chakras, which are related to survival, security, sensuality, sex and power, and the chakras above, related to a higher and more evolved consciousness.

The *anahata chakra* governs the sense of touch.

The *Vishuddhi Chakra* (Fifth Centre)

The Sanskrit word *shuddi* means 'to purify'.

Vishuddhi is the fifth chakra and is located in the cervical plexus, directly behind the base of the throat. It is symbolized as a violet or smoky purple-coloured lotus of 16 petals, corresponding to the number of *nadis* associated with this centre. Within the centre of the lotus is a downward-pointing triangle, containing a white circle, like the full moon, representing the element of ether (*akasha*) or space, which is more subtle than air.

On the physical level this chakra is related to the throat, neck, thyroid and parathyroid glands.

Vishuddhi is associated with the sense of hearing and is the centre for communicating, creativity, self-expression, and learning to accept and receive.

The *Ajna Chakra* (Sixth Centre)

The Sanskrit word *ajna* means 'to obey', 'to follow' or 'to know'. In the literal sense it means 'command centre'.

The *ajna chakra* is the sixth centre, located in the brain directly behind the space between the two eyebrows. It is linked to the pituitary gland.

THE SUBTLE BODIES AND THE CHAKRAS 17

Traditionally in yoga texts, the *ajna chakra* is symbolized by a two-petalled lotus, light grey in colour like a rainy day, or silvery-white like the moon. On the left petal is the Sanskrit letter *ham* and on the right *ksham*. These are the *bija* (seed) mantras for *shiva* and *shakti* (consciousness and energy). The left petal represents the moon (*ida nadi*) and the right petal the sun (*pingala nadi*). Inside the lotus is a circle with an inverted triangle, which represents *shakti* – creative energy and manifestation. Within the triangle is the *shivalingam*, not a phallic symbol but a symbol of the astral body. Above the *shivalingam* is the traditional symbol of *om*. This sound vibration is the *bija* mantra for this chakra.

Paramhansa Yogananda described the *spiritual eye*, which we can see during deep meditation, as a ring of gold light with an opalescent, violet-blue field within, and a five-pointed silvery-white star in the centre. Both the spiritual eye and the physical eye are reflections of the medulla oblongata (the base of the hind brain at the top of the spine). By concentrating on the point between the eyebrows (spiritual eye) one can see the medulla reflected as one light. This is the meaning behind Jesus Christ saying, 'If, therefore, thine eye be single, thy whole body shall be full of light.' (Luke 11:34–35)

The medulla oblongata is where the life-force (*prana*) primarily enters into the body. The *prana* is stored in the *sahasrara chakra* (seventh centre) and distributed throughout the whole body through the subtle network of nerve pathways (*nadis*). The medulla is also the seat of ego-consciousness, symbolized by the moon. The moon only reflects the sun's light, so the ego has no reality of its own, no light but that which it reflects from the soul.

What we need to do is transform ego-consciousness into soul-consciousness by deep and prolonged concentration at the spiritual eye, until the centre of consciousness becomes established at that point.

It is interesting to note that Lord Shiva is depicted with the moon symbol in his hair, in the *sahasrara chakra*, showing that his ego-consciousness is totally one with the cosmic Consciousness.

Sri Kriyananda said:

> The spiritual eye and the physical eye are reflections of the medulla oblongata, which is a cross-section of the spine itself and shows the various sheaths for the energy in the spine. There

are three concentric passages there. The outer passage is reflected in the spiritual eye as a ring of gold, and in the human eye as the white of the eye. This represents the energy world, the astral world. As you meditate deeply on it for many years, you will begin to see the spiritual eye elongate, and you will see a golden tunnel. As you go more deeply, you will see the blue field elongate into a tunnel. Going into that, you will go into the Christ Consciousness, which is also the causal world. The star in the centre represents the Kingdom of God beyond all creation

The main *nadis*, *ida*, *pingala* and *sushumna*, merge into one stream of consciousness from the *ajna chakra* and flow up to the highest centre of consciousness, the *sahasrara chakra*.

By meditating on this chakra one can gain intuitional knowledge and self-mastery, and destroy the *karma* of past lives.

The spiritual eye is the seat of will-power, so by concentrating at this point one can gain extraordinary will-power and spiritual strength.

The *Sahasrara* Chakra (Seventh Centre)

The Sanskrit word *sahasrara* means 1,000. It is for this reason that it is called the 1,000-petalled lotus. In fact, we cannot comprehend the magnitude of this vast lotus, with its infinite number of petals. It is said to be brighter and whiter than the full moon, tinged with the colours of the morning sun.

Sahasrara is also referred to as the crown chakra. It is the seventh and highest centre of consciousness, expanding above and beyond the six chakras below it. It is the store and distributing centre of power for them.

Sahasrara is the centre of divine union – when *kundalini shakti* ascends through the chakras and reaches *sahasrara*, the moment of self-realization or *samadhi* begins. The experience, the experienced and the experiencer become one and the same. The yogi experiences complete bliss in this superconscious state of *samadhi*. To reach this divine union in *sahasrara* we must first awaken the *ajna chakra*, which is the gateway to it. During deep meditation when the mind is concentrated at the spiritual eye (seen as a circular field of blue light, surrounded by a ring of gold light) a psychic passage opens up and connects the spiritual eye to the top of the head.

The Subtle Bodies and the Chakras 19

Until we awaken *ajna chakra* we remain in delusion, with our mind functioning within a limited sphere.

The *sahasrara chakra* is linked to the pineal gland.

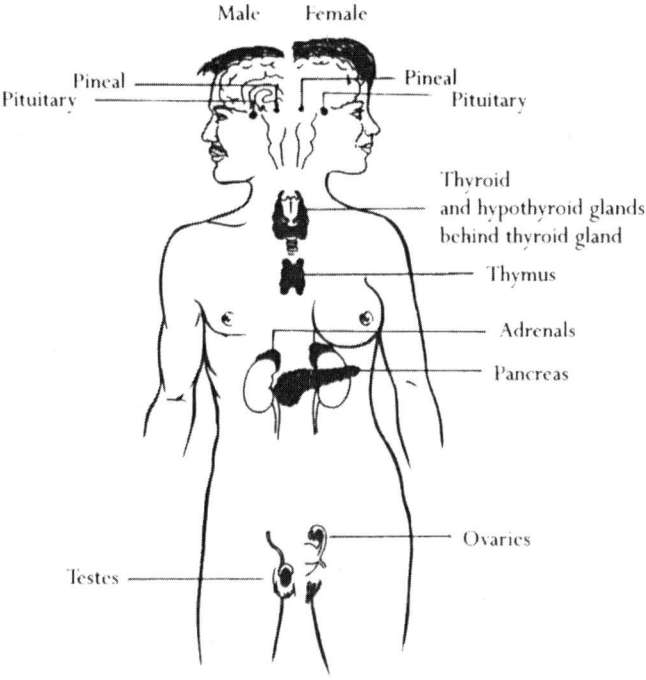

Figure 6 *The endocrine glands*

Gland	Chakra
Pineal	Sahasrara
Pituitary	Ajna
Thyroid	Vishuddhi
Thymus	Anahata
Pancreas	Manipura
Gonads and ovaries	Swadhisthana
Adrenals	Muladhara

Endocrine/Chakra Relationship

On the physical level each chakra is related to and has a significant effect on a ductless gland. The endocrine glands are ductless structures which secrete hormones directly into the circulation to regulate all the functions of the body (see figure 6).

When there is a balance between the astral and physical systems, the life-current energy becomes harmoniously connected and synchronized. However, if the flow of energy is blocked and imbalanced in the chakras, the corresponding endocrine gland will be affected, causing malfunction in the physical body, with mental and emotional changes.

Nerve Plexus/Chakra Relationship

The chakras are also related to the nerve plexuses, which are located along the physical spinal cord (see figure 7). Each nerve plexus is like a telephone exchange that receives and transmits nervous impulses and energy to the various body parts.

Locating the Chakras

The following is an exercise for locating your chakras.

Sit in a comfortable meditation posture with your spine upright and relax. If you are unable to sit with your legs crossed, then sit in an upright chair. It is important to keep your spine upright so that the energy can flow to the higher brain centres.

First, become aware of your astral spine by placing your left hand at the base of your spine and your right hand at the base of your skull (medulla oblongata). Close your eyes and calmly look into your spiritual eye (the point between your eyebrows). Inhale and feel your breath rising up from the base of your spine to the medulla oblongata. Exhale and feel the breath moving down through the astral spine. Practise 12 breaths.

Now place your left hand at your spiritual eye, while keeping your right hand at the medulla oblongata. As you inhale, feel the breath flow

THE SUBTLE BODIES AND THE CHAKRAS 21

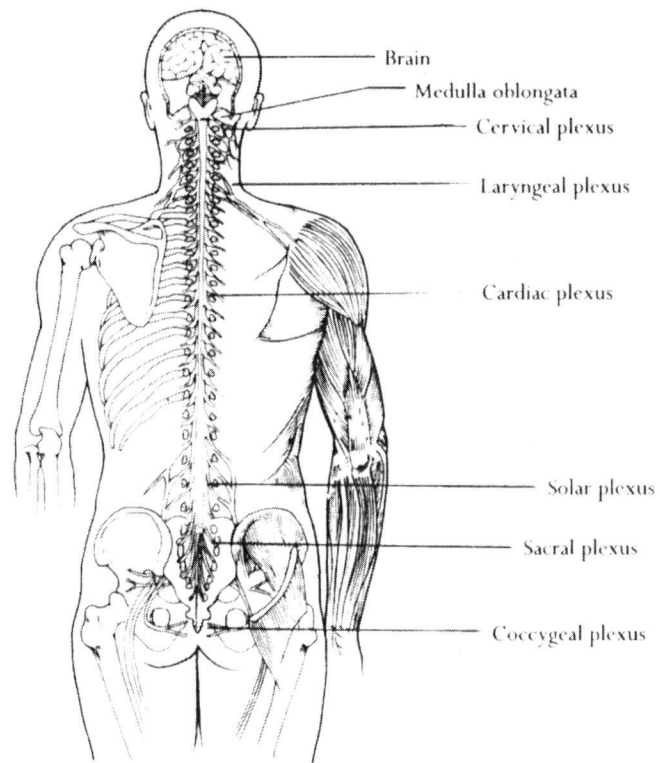

Rear view of spine – vertebrae and muscles cut away
showing spinal chord and spinal nerves

Figure 7 *The nerve plexuses*

Nerve Plexus	Chakra
Cavernous plexus	Ajna
Laryngeal plexus	Vishuddhi
Cardiac plexus	Anahata
Solar plexus	Manipura
Sacral plexus	Swadhisthana
Coccygeal plexus	Muladhara

through the psychic passage in the brain from the medulla to the spiritual eye. Exhale and feel your breath and energy flow from your spiritual eye to the medulla.

In the second part of this exercise we will contract and relax certain parts of the physical body, and visualize each chakra as a lotus flower.

Muladhara. Contract and relax the anus sphincter muscles. During contraction visualize a lotus with its petals closed and pointing downwards. Then visualize this lotus turning through 180 degrees so that it is pointing upwards, opening its petals. Now mentally chant '*om*' three times. Relax the contraction and direct the energy (the lotus rays of energy from the petals) up to the next chakra.

Swadhisthana. Contract and relax the sexual organs. Repeat as above, visualizing the lotus and mentally chanting '*om*' three times. Direct the energy up to the next chakra.

Manipura. Contract and draw the navel sharply in towards the spine and hold it there. Repeat the visualization and mental chanting as above and move the energy to the next chakra.

Anahata. Contract and pull the shoulders back. Repeat the lotus visualization and mental chanting as above and direct the energy up to the next chakra.

Vishuddhi. Stretch the neck backwards to feel a sensation in the throat. Repeat the visualization and mental chanting as before and move the energy to the next chakra.

Ajna. Concentrate deeply at the point between the eyebrows by turning the eyes upwards toward this point.

2

YAMA

ASHTANGA YOGA: THE EIGHT LIMBS OF YOGA

Patanjali, an ancient yogi-sage, integrated and simplified the science of yoga concisely in his *Yoga Sutras* during the 3rd century AD. These sutras can be considered as a collection of aphorisms on yoga. They are referred to as *The Yoga Sutras of Patanjali*, and are not the original exposition of a philosophy, but a compilation of work.

In them, he divided the path of Raja Yoga ('Royal Yoga', the king of yogas) into eight limbs, referred to as Ashtanga Yoga. These eight limbs give us an understanding of the deeper purposes and directions of yoga. They were devised by him to show us through yoga practice how to attain self-realization.

There is a misconception that Ashtanga Yoga consists of eight 'steps', but the word does not mean 'step'. *Ashta* means 'eight' and *anga* means 'limb'. In practising yoga, it is incorrect to isolate one limb and call that yoga. This is like a man's amputated arm telling you, 'I am John Smith,' when in fact, the arm is cut off from the main body and is nothing but a lump of dead flesh. One limb does not make a complete person.

Similarly, the yoga student who only practises yoga postures, ignoring the other limbs, such as *yama, niyama* and meditation, is not practising true yoga. Nor is meditation yoga without the practice of *yama* and *niyama*. Merely shifting emphasis from one limb to the other does not make one more essential than the other. Yoga is integration and wholeness; only the eight limbs practised together constitute yoga.

The eight limbs of yoga are:

1 *yama*: moral and ethical restraints – social discipline
2 *niyama*: observances – individual discipline
3 *asana*: posture, seat
4 *pranayama*: control of the life-energy through the breath
5 *pratyahara*: mind withdrawal from the senses
6 *dharana*: concentration
7 *dhyana*: meditation
8 *samadhi*: superconsciousness or union with the Divine

The eighth limb, called *samadhi* (superconsciousness) is not really considered a limb, because it *is* enlightenment or a state of union with the Divine.

We shall look at each of these limbs in turn in the following chapters, starting with *yama*.

THE RELATIONSHIP BETWEEN *YAMA* AND *NIYAMA*

Yama and *niyama* are divided into ten principles or ten commandments (without the Christian connotation of sin weighing heavily upon them). They are universal human practices, and are the foundation stones of all true religions.

The essential purpose of *yama* and *niyama* is to promote moral and ethical principles within the individual. They are an integral part of yoga practice and we cannot advance spiritually without practising them. They help to purify and steady the mind. Patanjali explains in Sutra 1:3 that when one has control over the mind and its modifications, one establishes oneself in one's true nature (the Self).

Yama and *niyama* have an intimate relationship – *niyama* safeguards *yama*. For example, if one has contentment (the *niyama santosha*) one will not steal (the *yama asteya* – 'non-stealing'), tell a lie (*satyam* – truth) or harm others (*ahimsa* – 'non-violence'). Another example is if one has internal purity (the *niyama saucha*), one can achieve chastity (*brahmacharya*).

THE PRINCIPLES AND PRACTICE OF *YAMA*

There are five principles which constitute *yama* (restraints and social disciplines). These are all interdependent and one needs to understand them in a subtle as well as in an obvious way.

The word *yama* means 'restraint' – self-restraint. *Yama* basically means 'to refrain' from actions, words and thoughts which cause distress and harm to others. Yama is also the name of the King of Death. In this context, *yama* means there must be a dying to ignorance, which is the source of egoism, attachment and repulsion.

The five principles of *yama* are: *ahimsa* (non-violence), *satya* (truth) *asteya* (non-stealing), *brahmacharya* (purity) and *aparigraha* (non-attachment) (*The Yoga Sutras of Patanjali* 2:30).

To purify and steady the mind, these restraints should be practised in thought, word and deed at all times, under all circumstances, wherever you are.

Patanjali instructs us to examine life and to see that all experiences that give temporary pleasure are tainted by sorrow and pain. He tells us that the cause of sorrow and pain is the identification of the seer (Self) with the seen (nature). When there is a unity of the seer (experiencer) and the seen (experienced) without the division of thought, then sorrow and pain do not arise.

Patanjali says, 'One can avoid sorrow and pain that has not yet manifested.' And how does one do that? By practising yoga: 'Yoga is the stilling of the movement of thought (without expression or suppression) in the undivided consciousness.' (*Yoga Sutras* 1:2)

All paths of yoga have the same goal – liberation of the mind from all obstacles to realizing the Self. Yoga is the dissolution of the psychological division within oneself, between what one *is* and what one wishes to be.

By examining your thoughts, words and actions with awareness and discrimination, you can come to an understanding of why problems and obstacles occur, and by which means they can be avoided. One practises yoga and meditation to remove the obstacles that stand between oneself and God. When the obstruction is removed, we have clear vision. What is the obstacle and how is it removed? By turning the attention within (Self-awareness) to observe the inner obstacles, thoughts and feelings, the obstruction will be revealed. You will realize what agitates the mind and veils the truth.

To obtain a greater awareness of the *yamas* and *niyamas,* and to bring the practice of them into your everyday life, begin by taking one *yama* or *niyama* each week. Keep a diary or notebook with you to record your observations. Observe with awareness, your own as well as that of others, your thoughts, words and actions in relation to the *yama* or *niyama* you are working with each week.

AHIMSA: NON-VIOLENCE, NON-INJURY, NON-HARMING

The goal of yoga is to realize that all life is one. If we are to truly live in that realization, we must affirm that oneness and unity by being kind, compassionate and respectful to all living beings in thought, word and actions.

We must refrain from causing or wishing harm, distress or pain to any living being, including ourselves and the environment. It would also be equally wrong to approve of another person's harmful or violent actions. Violence is very destructive at any level. We should not only refrain from violence against living beings, but against all forms — there can be violence in the way you close a door, in picking a rare wild flower or polluting the environment.

Ahimsa is not merely non-killing or 'Thou shalt not kill'. To live in *ahimsa*, it is important to develop an attitude of perfect harmlessness with positive love and respect for all life, not just in our actions, but in our thoughts and words as well. With perfect practice of *ahimsa* one rises above anger, hatred, aggression, fear, jealousy, resentment, envy and attachment. With perfection of *ahimsa* one realizes the unity and oneness of all life and attains universal love, peace and harmony.

THE PRACTICE OF *AHIMSA*

1 Make the mind steady and be even-minded.

Unsteadiness of the mind or restlessness is an obstacle to spiritual progress. In his sutras (2:3), Patanjali lists five afflictions that disturb mental equilibrium: ignorance (lack of spiritual knowledge), egotism, attraction to pleasure and aversion to pain, and clinging to life. Of these five afflictions, ignorance (*avidya*) is the source of all the other obstacles.

When one feels hatred, resentment, anger, jealousy or violence toward another, the mind and breath become unsteady. Abandon all destructive and negative thoughts; cultivate the opposite, positive qualities of love, compassion, patience, tolerance, sympathy and kindness.

Observe others when they become angry or harsh in their words and actions. Analyse their motives and behaviour. Observe your own thoughts, words and actions. Do you have thoughts that are self-destructive? Do you become defensive when criticized? When and why do you become angry? Where does this anger arise from?

2 Regularly practise self-inquiry.

Analyse your good and bad tendencies. Keep a spiritual diary and record in it at the end of the day your conduct, thoughts, words and actions. Be totally honest with yourself and make the necessary changes for improvement. Train your mind to think positive, inspiring thoughts.

3 Study the lives of those great souls who attained perfection in non-violence.

These include Mahatma Gandhi, St Francis of Assisi, Buddha, Jesus Christ, Paramhansa Yogananda and others.

4 Practise yoga *asanas* (see chapter 4), *pranayama* (see chapter 5) and meditation (see chapter 8) to control the body, breath and mind.

5 Meditate with love and devotion daily at the same time.

6 Pray for others and forgive them for their faults.

7 Give service to others and perform all your actions with love and awareness.

The Power of Affirmation

The first step towards Self-realization is bringing the mind into balance and harmony with the true Self. It is re-establishing our wholeness with life. This requires a self-education on our part: a self-awareness, an attentiveness to life from moment to moment.

The truth and reality remain hidden from us because we have identified our self with the mind, which has a limited vision of reality. It is only through wrong or false identification of the self with the mind that ignorance exists – 'I am this personality', 'this is mine', 'I am this body'. As soon as we drop this false idea and regain our true identity as pure consciousness, the Self (*Atman*), then ignorance and the ego of separateness disappear.

Our everyday thoughts, words and actions create our habits, desires, behaviours, emotions, attitudes, and sense-urges. These in turn shape and mould our life into the personality and character that we have made for ourselves.

When not established in Self-awareness, the soul is inclined to be identified with the mind and body-personality independent of our true spiritual nature.

On a day-to-day basis it is important to be aware and mindful of our thoughts, words and actions. *Awareness* is the key to the art of living. How many of us are aware that it is a blessing to be alive in a human form, where self-knowing and self-discovery is possible? If we are not aware of this sacred opportunity to relate to the life around us, we may equate the act of living only with going to school, acquiring a degree according to our talents, having a career, getting married or not married, bringing up the family, securing life with insurance policies and bank balances, repeating pleasures and sufferings, likes and dislikes – getting entangled in the mind-field of ego and continuing like this until old age, disease and finally death takes us away from this world.

Without ever truly knowing who we are and why we are here, we miss knowing what the true purpose of life is.

Our thoughts shape our destiny. We are what we think, not only consciously but also subconsciously. For years we have repeated words and statements, and attached meaning to them with our thoughts and feelings, which have created seed impressions in the soil of our subconscious mind. These impressions sink into the subconscious mind from the conscious mind and remain there, holding us in our conflicting patterns of feeling, habit and reaction.

The subconscious records all of what we think and believe, whether we want it or not. We give out the orders and the subconscious carries them out. Every act and every condition has its origin in the mind. Thoughts, whether positive or negative, are seeds that, when dropped or planted in the subconscious mind, germinate, grow and produce their fruit in due season.

The superconscious mind or intuitive mind works through the subconscious when the pathways of the subconscious are open. So, we must be careful to create positive pathways when we impress the subconscious mind.

To change the conflicting subconscious patterns of feeling and habit we can use the power of positive affirmation.

An affirmation is a statement of truth-positive words, that are repeated verbally and mentally for the purpose of confirming what is true, or of what we want to be true; or awakening to what is more desirable.

Affirmations are always worded to describe ideal circumstances as existing in the present. We affirm what *is*, not what we hope for.

Throughout this book there are affirmations to help you make positive changes in your life; they will help you to open to spiritual energy and awareness.

HOW TO USE AFFIRMATIONS

For affirmations to effectively help us, they need to be repeated consciously with awareness, with intensity of attention, with faith and conviction.

They should be repeated regularly throughout the day, for as many days or weeks until the desired result, change or awakening is attained.

The best time to practise is immediately after awakening in the morning, or at night, just before going to sleep. Other good times are after deep meditation and in quiet, relaxed periods when the mind is calm and more receptive to positive suggestions.

METHOD

1 Relax the body from tension and release the mind from anxiety, worry and restlessness. Breathe in deeply and tense your whole body while holding your breath for five seconds, then release the tension and exhale deeply. Repeat twice more.
2 Sit still in a comfortable meditation posture in which the head, neck and spine are held straight. Close the eyes and become aware of the natural breath flowing in and out. Practise this breath awareness for a few minutes or until the mind becomes calm.
3 When the body is still and the mind is calm and free from restlessness, then repeat your affirmation with deep concentration with the eyes closed, looking inwardly at the spiritual eye (the point between the eyebrows). Repeat your affirmation several times *loudly* to command the attention of your conscious mind. Then repeat it *quietly* to absorb the meaning more deeply. Continue to speak it very quietly, in a *whisper*. Then *mentally*, contemplating the meaning more intently as you gaze into the spiritual eye raising the consciousness toward superconsciousness.
4 After the practice session maintain awareness and inner calm. Establish the feeling within you that the condition you desire is already a part of your life. Visualize and know this to be true. With inner conviction, know, feel and visualize that your affirmations are working for you now!

Remember: An affirmation declares that which is true and opens the way for its manifestation.

Affirmation

Each day I become more consciously aware.

I remain vigilant against superficial differences and conflicts. I discriminate wisely. Instead of fault-finding, criticizing, judging and blaming others for seeming mistakes and deficiencies, I consider myself and others worthy of love, forgiveness and respect.

I see all people as expressions of the one Life. I am set free from limitation by the truth of my oneness with God. In this knowledge I walk the path of selfless love, knowing that there is no place for violence in love. Love is my divine nature and I have an endless capacity for love, which is ever seeking expression through me. God dwells within everyone's heart.

Satya: Non-lying, Truthfulness

To exaggerate, pretend, distort or lie to others, or to manipulate people for our own selfish concerns, is against our essential nature. Our essential nature is truth and living in truthfulness means to be anchored in the awareness of God.

Honesty with oneself is the first step to self-improvement. Without integrity in a relationship there can be no trust and without trust no credibility or mutual respect. Dishonesty is due to selfishness and the fear of a loss of reputation, to which one loses claim by being a hypocrite.

How can you ever achieve any success in self-realization or self-knowledge by sending out false messages about yourself? If you tell lies, you build up a personality which consists of lies and you deceive yourself. You can never know what truth is if you are immersed in lying.

To be truthful is not to be tactless. Thoughtfulness is essential to the usefulness of truth in relationship to others.

If you live in truth you will have peace of mind, free from fear, anxiety and worry. People will respect you from all walks of life. Those that live in truth have the power of the universe behind their thoughts and intentions.

THE PRACTICE OF *SATYA*

1 Introspect.

Search out truths about yourself on all levels, including your likes and dislikes, without being judgemental or prejudiced. Be ready to admit your faults and errors without feelings of guilt or sorrow, yet be sensitively aware of harm caused to others.

2 Develop an attitude of truthfulness.

Always recognize and accept the state of things and circumstances as they are and work with what *is*.

3 Be aware of your thoughts.

Only speak those words which are truthful. Before you speak, examine your thoughts to determine if they are selfish or harmful. Will they cause distress to someone? Your thoughts, words and actions should be in harmony.

4 Speak and observe the truth in thoughts, words and actions.

Do this even in circumstances where no one will stand by you.

5 Understand that God is Truth.

See God in everything and everyone. Truth promotes the welfare of all living beings and brings love, harmony and peace.

6 Observe silence and practise self-observation.

Silence is more than closed lips, the constant chattering of the mind also has to be stilled until there is an inner silence. To be still is to be in the presence of God. In the Bible (Psalm 46:10) it says: 'Be still and know that I am God.' In understanding this simple verse we can truly find inner communion with God. God cannot speak to our minds nor can He fill our hearts with inspiration when our consciousness is not attuned to the inner silence. Energy slowly gathers when the mind is silent. Thought and egoic preoccupations scatter the energy. When the mind is still, it reflects life accurately, without distortion.

When the mind is still, introspection and self-observation can take place. In this silence one becomes aware of the different types of thoughts; the sacred thoughts, the desires, the longings and the fears. Observe every thought and feeling as it arises in the mind, being aware of its cause, content and meaning. By observing your thoughts like this, suppressed experiences in the unconscious mind start to unfold themselves, releasing tremendous energy, while unburdening the unconscious mind of all conflict. After some time of practice the mind will experience a stillness in which there is no observer or observed, just awareness of silence and peace.

AFFIRMATION

I am now committed to purposeful living in order to clear my mind and consciousness. I contemplate only that which is good for me and good for others. I express truth in thought, word and deed to all living beings. I live in truth, love and harmony, and share it with others. I see the divine nature in every person I meet; love and goodwill continually flow out through me, thereby blessing them.

ASTEYA: NON-STEALING

The main reasons for people stealing are insecurity, selfishness, greed, a poverty consciousness and desperation.

Greed and desire are the source of stealing. Desire keeps one continually looking to the future for one's fulfilment, instead of realizing that perfection is attainable here and now. The mind is constantly turning outward, because it believes that fulfilment lies in the external world. To try to gain satisfaction by fulfilling the endless desires that arise in the mind is an utterly futile endeavour; it will only cause unhappiness and sorrow. Desire arises from the ego, from the thought of 'I', 'I want', 'I need', 'I must have'. Examine your desires and you will find that what you are really wanting or seeking is eternal happiness and joy, eternal peace, and eternal love. To experience this we must look within, it cannot be found outside of ourselves. Jesus says: 'The Kingdom of God is within you.' (Luke 17:2)

Once you attain love, joy and peace from within, it will also come to you from without.

It is through forgetfulness of our true identity and our relationship to God that we feel lost, experience unhappiness and live in a poverty consciousness. The Spirit of God dwells within us, but until we have a conscious awareness of God's presence within, it cannot bear fruit in our experience.

It is like forgetting our identity in sleep but recalling it on waking, when in fact it has never been lost.

When we are consciously aware, open to the universe, attuned and surrendered to God, life provides all that we need and more. God is the Consciousness from which we derive everything and we are all a part of that Consciousness. God is the source of all supply. He is the source of your very existence. We live only in our relationship to God – we are in God and God is in us. There is only one spiritual power – God is the Power, Source and Primal Cause. So instead of giving your power to outward circumstances, conditions and opinions of others, give all power to the Spirit within you. Eliminate all negative thoughts of lack, poverty and failure from your mind. Live more from within by attuning your will with God's Will, and let divine wisdom be your guide in everything.

Stealing out of necessity cannot be justified because it means violating another's right to keep what he or she has earned or inherited. *Asteya* means not depriving others of what belongs to them. In the case of someone who is homeless and steals a loaf of bread because they are hungry and have no money, the individual should be accountable for the crime first of all, while society should take the necessary measures to treat the cause.

People steal material objects from others, but stealing can also take place on a subtle level. We can steal people's time, affections, emotions, attentions, ideas and thoughts, to win attention and fame for ourselves.

Stealing also breaks the *yama* principles of truthfulness by lying and dishonesty to conceal the theft; non-violence because stealing disturbs the mind of the victim of theft; and non-attachment by stealing with greed. Hoarding too much of anything is also stealing.

The Practice of *Asteya*

1 Realize and understand that it is the desire or need for something apart from God that keeps us in separation from Him.

Misunderstanding leads us to believe that we can be satisfied with something outside of ourselves, other than the presence and the Power of God.

2 Channel all your desires into one desire – the desire for Self-awareness and Self-realization.

When you hold this desire above all others, the others will subside.

3 Develop a consciousness of abundance, so that you are able to receive freely from the universal supply.

Realize that if you have any sense of lack, it is because your thoughts, ideas and beliefs have conditioned your mind to think that way. Turn your thoughts from lack and limitation to the belief in the inevitable law of God working for you in abundance. Attune your will to God's Will and visualize yourself as you want to be. Retain that image and sustain it joyfully with faith and expectancy until you succeed in its attainment.

4 Give service to others.

Service awakens compassion and takes attention away from our personal feelings of lack. When we consciously serve and give from the heart, inner grace becomes operative in our lives.

5 Simplify your life by eliminating all non-essential things and activities.

This may also include associating with egocentric people who have conflicting and negative patterns of thought to your spiritual views on life.

YAMA   35

6 Break the habit of lack and limitation.
Cultivate higher states of consciousness and oneness with God by communing with God in deep meditation regularly.

AFFIRMATION

I am an individualized expression of God. God is my life. I am a channel through which God's abundance, love, peace, joy, health, power and intelligence ceaselessly and freely flow. Because I am made in the image of God, all that God has is embodied within my consciousness. God alone is the Divine Source. He is Infinite, and in my oneness with God I am thankful that I have everything I need. I take responsibility for my thoughts, attitudes and actions. I act and live honestly and express my highest spiritual self to the world.

BRAHMACHARYA: NON-SENSUALITY

Brahmacharya is the sum and substance of yoga and literally means, 'when the inner consciousness flows constantly towards Truth, the Absolute (Brahman)'. It also means purity in thought, word and action.

In India, some yogis and swamis restrict its meaning by interpreting *brahmacharya* as restraint of the sex impulse or celibacy, rather than as a sublimation of passion through deeper emotions of loving, kindness and affection. If *brahmacharya* only meant celibacy then married people who wanted children would not be able to practise yoga. *Brahmacharya* has a wider meaning than the restraint of the sex impulse, otherwise there could not have been householder saints with children. One such saint was Lahiri Mahasaya who was initiated into the ancient technique of Kriya Yoga by the immortal master Mahavatar Babaji in the foothills of the Himalayas in 1861. Lahiri Mahasaya and his wife had five children born to them some years after Lahiri's initiation by Babaji.

It is interesting to note that in ancient times many saints were householders. They would bring up families while continuing their practice of yoga and leading a spiritual life. To them, there was no conflict between sex and God. It was only later that asceticism and celibacy entered into the Indian religious tradition.

In most religious traditions sexuality is regarded as an obstacle to spiritual life, which has ingrained in the human consciousness feelings of guilt, shame and having sinned.

Sexuality in itself is neither pure nor impure, it only becomes impure if it is used without discrimination, understanding, respect, care, love and responsibility. There is nothing to be ashamed or guilty about, for we would not be here without it. God created sex for the purposes of procreation and creativity, not for sense-gratification and selfish pleasure.

RELATIONSHIP AND SEXUALITY

Brahmacharya is not the abandonment of sex, but the transcendence of it. The question is not, 'Shall I renounce sex, marriage and social responsibility for a life of spiritual practice?', but 'What is the right relationship to them?' Whether one is following the householder's path or the path of renunciation, the question is the same.

From a spiritual or moral point of view, a sexual relationship is not dependent on being married or not, but on *commitment*. There has to be commitment, responsibility, care, love and concern for each other to make the relationship meaningful. Otherwise it is a relationship of possessing an object for ego-gratification through the senses. Sexuality is *not* just a toy provided for our physical pleasure divorced from love, commitment, care and responsibility.

Love can express itself naturally and spontaneously in joyful sexual intimacy without feelings of guilt or shame. But if your relationship with another is based on self-gratification, you will find that you disregard the feelings of that partner and sooner or later the relationship is destroyed. For a true relationship to form, the identification of others as objects for self-gratification must end.

If we are attached to the goal of orgasm then sex becomes an addiction, and like any other addiction our mind becomes preoccupied with it, causing us tension. Excessive indulgence in sensuality causes pain and sorrow. The mind becomes agitated; the intellect is impaired and one is not able to discriminate. One's physical radiance and magnetism decreases with loss of energy and vitality; boredom, depression and discontent set in.

There is a fine balance between indulgence and abstinence. Repression or denial can be just as harmful as indulgence – both can be ego-orientated; both can make the mind dull, losing its sensitivity and awareness. There is no lasting joy in either indulgence or repression.

THE PRACTICE OF *BRAHMACHARYA*

1 Practise introspection and self-enquiry.

Ask yourself, 'Where does the experience of desire arise from? Did this desire, action or experience arise from the ego-sense or from my true Self, the soul intelligence within? Why has this thought or desire entered my mind? Whom does it concern? Who am I?

If you practise this Self-enquiry constantly and persistently, eventually all thoughts will drop away, and the ego will disappear. Only by understanding the nature of desires can you prevent them. By turning the mind inward to investigate its own source and nature, it is illuminated by Self.

When our mind is turned outward and lost in desires and attachments, our true eternal nature, Self, is forgotten. We have forgotten our true identity through over-identification with the body, mind and ego. We experience happiness and unhappiness, pleasure and pain because the body and mind are subject to change. That which changes cannot be real, only that which is permanent and eternal is real.

We must understand how 'I', the ego, got caught up in this conflict between what is and what is desired. The desire to experience creates the 'I'. If the desire to experience is absent, there is no ego-sense – what remains is pure experiencing. To some extent we can use the example of sleep. In deep sleep one can remain totally absorbed and integrated in the state in which one simply is, without a desire or craving for any other state. In sleep you become one with the state of sleep. There is no division and no pain. You do not experience sleep, nor do you desire to wake up. Sleep and 'I' are one – I am asleep, but I do not know I am asleep. I am sleeping peacefully and happily, but I do not know that. In the experience of sleep there is pure experience, no thought of 'I' or 'me', but when I awake from sleep the craving to experience arises again and it identifies itself as the 'I' or 'me'. This is the first thought that arises, then the 'I' thought connects itself to the other thoughts and casts a shadow of ignorance around itself. Thought is always a movement away from what is, it is a movement between the past and the future. When attention is distracted and diverted from our centre of awareness, we become divided. Conflict arises and our energy is scattered.

Yoga is being calmly centred within, in a state of attentive awareness at all times. In this state of awareness the mind is quiet, free from conflict.

2 Follow the middle path.

In the *Bhagavad Gita* (6:16–18) Lord Krishna advises us to follow the path of moderation.

> Yoga is not for those who eat too much or who eat too little, nor for those who sleep too much or sleep too little. But to those that are moderate in eating, sleeping, wakefulness, recreation and moderate in all their actions, yoga will bring an end to all sorrow. Those souls who have learned to discipline their mind and remain calmly established in the self, free from attachment to all desires, attain the state of union.

3 Transform your sexual energy.

> Sex pleasure dissipates one's energy in direct proportion to the consciousness of self-indulgence. When there is self-giving love, there is to some extent an upward flow of energy in the spine, and thus an inflow of divine energy in the form of love. It is not repression, however, when a person seeks with understanding to redirect the flow of this energy upward toward the brain. Energy so directed can give one tremendous powers of accomplishment on all levels of life. Where there is consent of the will there is not repression, but transmutation.

Sri Kriyananda, *14 Steps to Joy*

Through the practice of yoga and meditation the sexual energy (semen) on the physical level can be transmuted into spiritual or subtle energy (*ojas*) by directing and channelling it upwards, towards the higher brain centres, through the subtle pathway in the spine called the *sushumna*. This energy is then stored in the brain as *ojas shakti*.

Both men and women have vital fluids whose loss due to excessive sexual indulgence causes loss of vitality and unsteadiness of *prana* in the body. For obvious reasons the man loses more of this vital fluid during the sexual act than the woman does.

Those who are following a spiritual path and are not married or in a sexual relationship will find the following yoga postures and practices beneficial in conserving and transforming the seminal energy on the physical level into *ojas shakti* on the spiritual level.

Those people who are married or in a sexual relationship can also gain benefit from these practices, for they have rejuvenating and toning effect on the glands, nerves, sex centre and body systems, promoting and prolonging youth and vitality.

- *Siddhasana* (adept's pose) (see chapter 8). This meditative seated posture prevents the formation of semen by acting on the testes and its cells. It also pushes *prana* into the *sushumna*.

- *Sarvangasana* (shoulder stand). Prevents nocturnal discharges and helps to directs the flow of seminal energy towards the brain.
  1. Lie flat on your back with a blanket folded in two under your shoulders to protect your neck. Align your neck, spine and legs in a straight line.
  2. Bend your knees with your feet on the floor. *Inhale* and raise your hips off the floor, supporting them with your hands.
  3. *Exhale* as you bring your hands to your back and drop your knees to rest on your forehead. Bring your elbows closer together.
  4. Inhale and extend your trunk upwards, tucking your chin into your collarbone. Exhale while raising your hips and thighs until your knees point to the ceiling or sky.
  5. Inhale, extend your trunk, and tighten your buttocks as you straighten your legs, pulling them up from the hips, lifting as high as possible.

6   While holding the pose relax your buttocks, legs, feet, throat and facial muscles. Breathe normally. Hold the pose for 30 seconds. Advanced students can increase the time to five minutes.
7   To come out of the pose slowly lower your feet to a 45-degree angle over the head. Lower your arms to the floor behind your back, with your palms resting on the floor.
8   With control lower your back, vertebra by vertebra, to the floor until you are lying flat on your back.
9   Relax in *shavasana* (corpse pose – see page 132) for two or three minutes while concentrating on your breath.

Limitations
Do not practise if you:
- suffer from enlarged thyroid gland
- suffer from liver, spleen or heart ailments
- suffer from high blood pressure
- are menstruating

Stop your practice if you have pressure in the eyes or ears.

- **Sirshasana** (headstand). Helps to direct the flow of seminal energy towards the brain and prevents nocturnal discharges.
    1   Begin from *shashankasana* (pose of a child) – sit on your heels with your forehead resting on the floor, with your hands relaxed and palms upwards by your sides. Relax for a few moments in this pose.
    2   Kneel with your head firmly and comfortably resting on a folded blanket. Place your elbows shoulder-width apart. Bring your hands into a clasped position by interlocking the fingers against the back of your head. Rest the centre of the crown of your head on the blanket between your forearms.
    3   Raise your hips and walk your feet towards your head with your hips up and your knees straight.
    4   Bend your knees in towards your chest as you raise your feet from the floor, bringing your heels to your buttocks.
    5   With your back straight and your knees bent, slowly straighten your hips until your knees in their folded position are pointing towards the ceiling.
    6   Straighten your legs into the final position.

7 Come out of the pose slowly and carefully by bending your knees and drawing them into your chest. Gradually lower your feet to the floor and relax in the child's pose (*shashankasana*) again for a few seconds until breathing returns to normal.

Limitations
Do not practise if you:
- suffer from high blood pressure
- suffer from arthritis of the neck
- suffer from glaucoma
- are four or more months pregnant
- are menstruating

- **Padangushthasana** (toe-balance pose). The pressure of the heel on the perineum (the area between the anus and sexual organs) acts on the spermatic duct, and so prevents the external flow of semen and nocturnal discharges, and tones the reproductive glands.
  1 Kneel down and balance on your toes.
  2 Sit on your right heel and place your left foot on your right thigh in half lotus.
  3 Place your palms together at your chest.
  4 Concentrate on the tip of your nose. Inhale and hold your breath while balancing. Exhale and repeat on the opposite side.

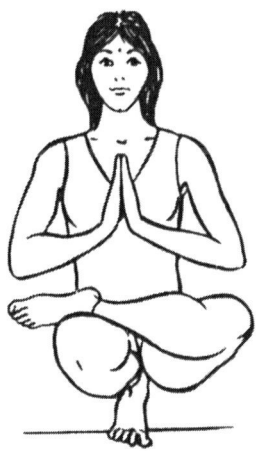

Figure 8 *Padangushthasana (toe-balance pose)*

- ***Viryastambhanasana*** (semen-retention pose). Helps counter the effects of sexual excesses. An effective posture for the sublimation of the sex urge. Strengthens the reproductive glands.
  1. Stand with your feet wide apart and clasp your hands behind your back; inhale.
  2. *Exhale*, bend your right knee so it forms a right angle to the floor. Keeping your back straight lower your trunk down on the inside of your right leg until your nose or forehead touches your right foot, the left leg is kept straight.
  3. Hold your breath for as long as comfortable while holding the pose, without strain.
  4. *Inhale* as you slowly rise out of the pose and stand erect and relax.
  5. Repeat on other side.

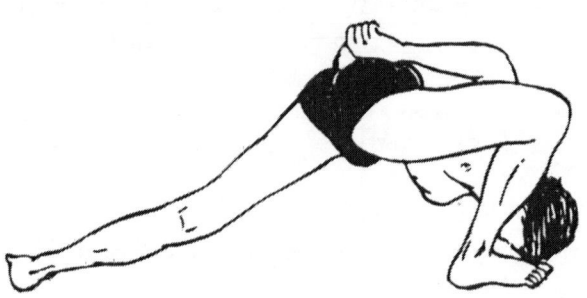

Figure 9 *Viryastambhanasana (semen-retention pose)*

- ***Matsyasana*** (fish pose). Tones up all the areas of the spine and the reproductive glands. It is particularly beneficial to women as it normalizes uterine functioning.
  1. Lying flat on your back bring your feet together, with your arms by your sides palms down.
  2. Slide your arms beneath your body, with your palms flat on the floor, so that you are sitting on your hands.
  3. With the weight of your body on the elbows inhale, lift your head and arch your lower back, raising your chest.
  4. Lower your head to the floor, so that the crown of your head is resting on the floor.
  5. Pushing with your elbows, arch your chest as high as possible. Feel your chest expanding. Breathe abdominally.

6   To come out of the position keep your body weight on your elbows, and lift your head and neck first before lowering your back down to the floor slowly as you exhale. Relax in *shavasana* (corpse pose).

- **Bandhas** (energy locks). These help in transmitting sexual energy to the higher energy centres, and control the movement of pranic energy. The *bandhas* are:
  - *mulabandha* ('root' or anal lock)
  - *uddiyana bandha* (diaphragm lock)
  - *jalandhara bandha* (chin lock)
  - *mahabandha* (triple lock)

There are also some *mudras* (energy seals) that are helpful in controlling the pranic energy – these in particular:

- **ashwini mudra** (gesture of the horse), a powerful technique for pumping the energy up into the third energy centre (*manipura chakra*)
- **viparita karani mudra** (reverse-posture *mudra*). Preserves the subtle nectar (*amrita*) that flows from the *sahasrara chakra*, promoting vitality and energy. This is an important practice for the sumblimation of sexual energy to the higher centres. (see chapter 4 for the technique)
- **vajroli mudra** (the thunderbolt), in which the muscles used to stop the flow of urine are contracted; after some practice a man can retain the energy from the semen even when ejaculating, transmitting it to the higher brain centres

The techniques for practising these bandhas and mudras are given in chapter 4.

- **Bhadrasana** (nobility pose). This posture is recommended for women, because it helps regulate the menstrual cycle. It also tones and strengthens the reproductive glands. It prevents nocturnal emissions in men.
  1   Sit on the floor and bring the soles of your feet together. Clasp your hands firmly around your feet and pull your heels in close to your sexual organs. Lift your chest and straighten your neck.

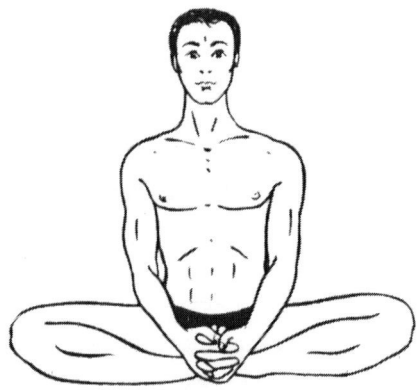

Figure 10 *Bhadrasana (nobility pose)*

2 Inhale slowly, pressing your knees and your thighs gently towards the ground, with your head, neck and spine in a straight line.
3 Hold your breath comfortably for ten seconds while concentrating on the energy flowing upwards to the spiritual eye (*ajna chakra*).
4 Slowly exhale and release the pose. *Note:* In the more advanced posture bend forward from the hips and bring your chin to the floor in front of your feet.

- **Gomukhasana** (cow's-head pose). Helps in sublimating the sex urge.
  1 Sit with your right leg crossed over your left, so your right knee sits above your left. Draw your feet backwards to rest beside your hips. This pose is called *virasana*.
  2 Raise your right arm over your right shoulder. Catch hold of your right hand by bringing your left hand behind your back.
  3 Inhale and stretch your shoulders and arms by pulling up with your right arm and down with your left.
  4 Hold your breath in the final pose.
  5 Slowly exhale, reverse your legs and arms and repeat the practice.

- **Pranayama** (control of the life-energy through the breath). By the practice of *pranayama* one controls the breath (the external manifestation of *prana*, life-force) and vital forces of the body. The mind, *prana* and semen have an intimate link. If one controls *prana*, then the mind is controlled. By controlling the seminal energy, the mind and *prana* are brought under control (see chapter 5 for the techniques).

4 Discriminate

Remember, happiness or pleasure is not in the objects you desire, but within your own Self (soul nature).
Study these words from the *Bhagavad Gita* (2:62–5).

> From thought comes attachment. From attachment desire arises. When desire is frustrated by an obstacle, anger springs up.
>
> When there is anger, one becomes easily deluded and loses memory of right and wrong. Loss of memory then leads to loss of discrimination. From this loss of intelligence, spiritual life is wasted.
>
> But those who can supervise the involvement between the senses and sense-objects by exercising self-control and who become free thereby from craving and from false repression attain inner calmness, in which all sorrows end. Then one soon becomes established in the Self.

5 Remember God first.

In the Bible we read: 'Seek ye first the Kingdom of God and His righteousness and all these things will be given to you' (Matthew 6:33) We do not have to look far to find the Kingdom of God. 'The Kingdom of God is within you.' (Luke 17:21)
   Through deep meditation with the consciousness calm and inwardly focused we can experience the presence of God in that inner silence. 'Be still and know that I am God.' (Psalm 46:10)
   Pray for God's grace and presence to be established in you. Realize your oneness with God for fulfilment in life.

6 Meditate regularly and deeply every day.

Meditation transcends egocentric thought processes, feelings and desires. Through meditation we can realize and express that pure consciousness, the reflection of God within us.

Your daily appointment with the Infinite during meditation is the most important time of the day.

7 Acknowledge the divine nature of others.

See others as spiritual beings and relate to them accordingly. See through all outer appearances; everyone has the same innate nature and potential for awakening and spiritual growth.

AFFIRMATION

God is the true source of contentment and fulfilment in my life. I rise above feelings of ego need and lack of any kind.

I find true fulfilment in God. I experience the love, peace, joy and harmony of God now. Whatever is necessary to my fulfilment will come into my experience by being consciously one with God. I remain open to the flow of God's grace in my life. Divine intelligence gives me the wisdom and guidance I need to achieve true joy and inspires me to right thought and right action. I neither repress nor pursue sensuality, but I follow the middle path by using my energy wisely. I channel it into true love, positive attitudes and for the purpose of higher consciousness. I remain responsible, caring and loving. I live each day in the complete awareness of God's reality within.

APARIGRAHA: NON-ATTACHMENT, NON-GREED

The Sankskrit word *apara* means 'of another' and *agraha* 'to crave for'. *Aparigraha* means 'without craving for what belongs to another'. It can also mean 'not hoarding or accumulating'.

The difference between non-covetousness and non-greed is that non-covetousness means not to desire what is not rightfully one's own, and non-greed means not to be attached even to what already *is* one's own.

People who act from attachment manipulate situations and other people because they fear that they will lose the desired object. Such people have no security in life because they are ruled by selfish desire, anger, greed and fear.

The problem arises when the mind clings to what one thinks one's security is derived from – 'My whole life depends upon that person', 'My security comes from being in this job, owning this house and being with my family.' We develop a false sense of security by placing our power in such transitory things or by accumulating more possessions than we actually need. There is no need to keep or strive to possess anything beyond the basic requirements for a comfortable life.

Security is not possible when there is fear, which is the first product of duality and division. Your true security is in God. He is always with you, within your heart. Let the Spirit of God move into every area of your life. Keep the spirit of truth alive in your heart and mind. With God, you cannot fail.

Security is the love in your heart. Your generosity and your capacity to give is your security. Give unconditionally, because when you give with conditions, they will return to you.

Your security in relationships is to love unconditionally, not demanding love in return. It is the nature of the heart to give love and once anything goes out of the heart, it is not lost because it is reflected back to you.

THE PRACTICE OF *APARIGRAHA*

1 Understand that everything belongs to God.

We came into this world without anything, and we will leave it without taking anything with us. There is not one thing or person that we truly own. We are only the caretakers of what is available to us, and we need to be responsible for its right use in life. This natural law applies to material possessions, relationships, environment and nature.

2 Purify the heart.

Purity of heart, right motivation and corresponding effort, not expecting something for which one has not worked or inherited, are the means to counter covetousness. Purify the heart of envy and jealousy.

3 Remember that God is the life of all.

If we continually give back to life without any selfish motive, the universe gives freely back to us.

4 Do not treat others as you yourself would not want to be treated.

5 Be aware that God is the true source of all our needs.

Jesus says:

> Take no thought for your life, what you will eat; or about your body, what you will wear. Life is more than food, and the body more than clothes. Consider the ravens: they do not sow or reap ... and God feeds them ... Consider the lilies how they grow: they toil not, they spin not. Yet I tell you, not even Solomon in all his splendour was dressed like one of these.
>
> (Luke 12:22–27)

He then goes on to say:

> Your Father knows that you need these things. But seek his Kingdom and these things will be given to you as well.
>
> (Luke 12:30–31)

Lord Krishna gives a similar parallel in the *Bhagavad Gita:*

> To those who worship Me alone, and constantly meditate on Me, without any other thought, I provide all their needs and give full security.
>
> Bhagavad Gita, 9:22

When we open ourselves to God by attuning our will to His Will, and remember Him, we receive His grace in greater abundance. By having faith in God and an understanding of divine grace, one can live a more fulfilling life.

6 Let go, let God.

Let go of attachment to those things, relationships, bad habits, negative attitudes and conditionings which block your awareness to higher understanding and Truth. Let go to let God's higher wisdom and grace be active in your life. Strength and understanding may not come all at once, but as we prove our desire for Truth is real, as we are willing to follow and trust, God will show us the way.

AFFIRMATION

I accept life and whatever life gives me.

I trust God, and my faith assures me that I am safe and secure. Wherever I am, God is, and I am protected.

The freedom, strength and security I need come from the sure knowledge that I am not alone. The spirit of God is with and within me, and I can always be more than I have ever before expressed.

I release all attachments to actions and the results of actions.

I let go of negative attitudes and conditionings which are not useful to higher understanding.

I am set free from all limitation and poverty consciousness by the truth of my oneness with God. Because the universe gives freely, I selflessly give to life in return. I know that the love I give expression to is from God, and God's supply of love is infinite.

My love, inner peace and ever-new joy is always secure when I am consciously aware and united with God's loving and guiding presence within.

3

NIYAMA

There are five principles of *niyama*: *saucha* (cleanliness, purity); *santosha* (contentment); *tapas* (austerity); *svadhaya* (self-study); and *isvarapranidhana* (surrender to God).

SAUCHA: CLEANLINESS, PURITY

When perfect cleanliness (purity of mind and body) is obtained, there arises a sense of detachment and transendence from the physical body, and a disinclination for contact with the bodies of others (seeking pleasure from others).

The Yoga Sutras of Patanjali 2:40

As a result of inner purity one experiences purification of the heart, inner peace, cheerfulness, power of concentration, mastery over the senses and the ability and qualification to attain self-realization.

ibid 2:41

Saucha means total cleanliness internally and externally. It means practising purity in thought, word and action. Purity on all levels frees the mind from its limitations.

The inner light of the soul within you is the same light in all people, but it appears to shine more brightly in some people than others. If you have two oil-burning lamps that give the same amount of light, but the glass window of one lamp is covered with dust and soot, then the other lamp will shine more brightly. It is not a matter of more light, but of cleaning or clearing away the impurities that are blocking the light. To allow the soul's light within us to shine freely and brightly we need to cleanse our physical body both internally and externally; purify our mind and emotions, and keep the environment in which we live clean and orderly.

Internal purity is more important than external purity, because when the mind is pure and one-pointed, one is able to see clearly and purely. Without cleanliness and purity (*saucha*), *brahmacharya* cannot be attained. *Brahmacharya* and *saucha* work together.

THE BODY AS A TEMPLE

'God's temple is holy, and that temple you are.' (1 Corinthians, 3: 17) The body is the temple of the soul. The soul within your body-temple is your essential nature, it is pure consciousness, eternal, immortal, an individualized expression of God Himself. We are spiritual beings made in the image and likeness of God!

We are born into this body-temple for a certain lifespan to experience a conscious relationship with God and to do God's Will. We then vacate the body, when it has served its purpose, and move into a new body (reincarnate).

Our purpose on earth, living in a human body, is to awaken in God-realization, to expand our consciousness from the human condition to God-consciousness, to be self-complete in God, and to inspire and assist others to grow spiritually. We need clearly to understand and define our life's purposes, then to become motivated and committed to them, until we experience and actualize our goal. To achieve this aim we need to expand our awareness, put our life in order, attend to our spiritual and purification practices, meditate regularly and give selfless service, live in harmony with nature's laws and be surrendered to God, Life and Grace.

We are the caretakers of our bodies for the duration of this lifetime. If through ignorance, laziness and lack of discipline the body becomes weak, disabled or diseased, with little or no energy, then it becomes an obstacle and distraction to the mind. When the mind is distracted it is very difficult to meditate, awareness is clouded and one is unable to see or think clearly.

When we see clearly and purely, the reality of God is radiated through us. Without clear perception our true reality, our soul-consciousness and awareness, and our relationship to the reality of God is coloured by our mental conditionings, habits, emotions and misguided desires. This results in our thoughts, behaviour and actions being determined by ignorance.

The Practice of *Saucha*

Physical Cleanliness

We need to re-educate our bodies and try to discover their original sensitivity by cleansing them of their accumulations of obstructions and impurities.

1 Avoid excessive use of intoxicants and stimulants.

Excessive use of intoxicants and stimulants such as drugs, smoking, alcohol, tea, coffee, meat, sugar, salt, strong spices and overloading the stomach with excess food brings about degeneration of the body organism and premature ageing, dulls the mind and sensitivity and makes it impure.

Medical opinion is unanimous on the point that *smoking* is harmful. It is bad for the heart, circulation, lungs, digestion, throat and the skin. Tobacco smoke has many dangerous chemicals – some of the more hazardous include tar, arsenic, carbon monoxide, nitrogen dioxide, ammonia, benzopyrene and hydrogen sulphide. Just think, a person who smokes a packet of non-filtered cigarettes a day for ten years, inhales approximately eight quarts of tar!

The yogi sees that tobacco is in no way helpful or beneficial to human health. In no way does it glorify God or the self in the body of the user. The yogi sees that not only do tobacco smokers harm themselves, but they also contribute negatively to the health and welfare of their fellow beings around them (breathing in second-hand smoke makes one a 'passive smoker').

Alcohol dries up the stomach's secretions and exhausts the liver and kidneys. It is also harmful to the nervous system and depletes the body's vitamin B and C supplies. It also overloads the enzyme system, leaving the body prey to free radicals. A free radical is an atom or group of atoms with an uneven electrical charge. To make itself complete, it steals a charged particle (electron) from a neighbouring cell, which sets off a chain of reactions producing more free radicals, damaging more cells. Alcohol also dehydrates the body's cells, interfering with their protein, causing premature cell death.

From a spiritual viewpoint, it is not the temporary intoxication that alcohol may induce, nor the hangover that sometimes follows, but the long-term effect that alcohol exerts on the personality. In some subtle way it seems to make one more worldly; one's perceptions become less refined, and one may even deride or ridicule things formerly considered sacred. The ego, in becoming less sensitively responsive to its environment, becomes more self-assertive and aggressive. Everyone should know deep within that drunkenness is an insult to their true divine nature.

A *drug*-based or drug-dependent reality is a chemical illusion, rather than the release and freedom which comes spontaneously out of an attentive observation and awareness of life, inner as well as outer.

One of the most important differences between the two kinds of experience (drug-induced bliss and true spiritual experience without drugs) is that the ecstasy of drugs fades – one goes up then comes down with a bang. It is bliss without true knowledge and vision. A true spiritual, mystical experience changes one's life, as can be seen from the lives of saints and sages.

Can we say that a drug addict has ever made a positive major contribution to mankind? It is the difference between the effects of truth and the effects of illusion. Often the basic philosophy and way of life of a person who has taken a few LSD trips are unaffected, or there may be a large discrepancy between his or her everyday life and the revelations whilst under the influence of the drug. Yet one who has a true spiritual mystical experience cannot remain unaffected. His or her life is influenced for the good by the deep inner convictions given by that knowledge.

When one takes drugs, deterioration of the mental faculties may begin to take place and become progressive. The intellect becomes impaired, judgement and discrimination fail. The attempts to transcend the ego fail, and one is in fact thrown back into the ego with all its associated sufferings.

On the other hand, the attainment of the highest spiritual state leads to complete mastery of the mind and mental faculties. Inspiration, intuitive insight and deep understanding develop. All the mental potentialities are fulfilled, for the light behind the mind, the soul within, is allowed to shine through unhindered.

Meat, fish and *eggs* should be avoided. A vegetarian diet is essential for one who wants to follow a spiritual life; if you wish to progress and grow from the ordinary and materialistic life to a higher spiritual life, then it becomes important to live on a vegetarian diet. Vegetarian foods help the mind and body become more refined; they help to calm the mind and body of their restlessness.

Purification of the body goes hand in hand with spiritual awakening. A vegetarian diet helps us in the purifying of the body and mind. It is highly conducive to sublime thoughts, divine contemplation, meditation and compassion. It renders the intellect keen, subtle and sharp, and gives greater vitality than animal food.

Meat is high in saturated fats containing cholesterol that accumulates on the arterial walls, constricting the flow of blood in the body, placing a greater burden on the heart to pump harder. Cholesterol is a major factor in causing heart attacks.

Meat-eaters' intestinal flora is changed from fermentative to putrefactive bacteria in the long bowel, causing poisons to be absorbed into the bloodstream. Toxic wastes from the dead animal's bloodstream, along with germs, antibiotics and drugs that have been injected into them to control the animal's diseases, contaminate our own blood when we eat meat.

Animal food, salt, sugar, tea, coffee and hot spices all dull the sensitivity of the nervous system if taken in excess.

In fact, indulgence to excess of any habit-forming pleasure dulls the sensitivity of the nervous system. If you really want to heighten your sensitivity and progress spiritually, sooner or later you will come to a point where you will have to give up these indulgences or habits. Sensory pleasure beyond a certain point becomes self-defeating. If you continually indulge in pleasures like smoking, drinking or taking drugs, sooner or later the pleasure will ruin the mind and destroy the body.

2 Practise yogic purifying techniques.

We can purify the body by regulating and disciplining our habits and by using yogic techniques of purification.

Cleanse the body internally through the practice of the *shat kriyas* (see chapter 4), periodic fasting and living on a pure vegetarian, wholefood diet.

NIYAMA 55

Externally, the body can be kept clean by bathing regularly and thoroughly (see chapter 4 on how to clean the body).

The practice of *yoga asanas* (yoga postures – see chapter 8) promotes excellent health and vitality; they tone, revitalize and strengthen the whole physical organism. Yoga postures remove toxic physical impurities, tension and obstructions to the flow of energy in the body. Through the practice of *yoga asanas* the internal organs are maintained in a healthy functioning order; the blood and lymphatic systems circulate more freely; *prana* (vital force) is distributed evenly throughout the body and its systems; the body is kept supple and the skeletal system is aligned in its correct position; one takes on a youthful appearance and life is extended.

The practice of *pranayama* (see chapter 5) gives lightness to the body and cleanses the subtle pathways (*nadis*). *Pranayama* nourishes all the body's tissues and cells with pure blood and lymph, the metabolism is improved and balanced and concentration is improved. By regular practice of *pranayama* the yogi stores a large supply of energy (*prana*), giving him or her strength and vitality. *Pranayama* also helps to purify and control the mind.

Mental Cleanliness

When the mind is purified one naturally experiences peace, cheerfulness, goodness of mind, the power of concentration, mastery over the senses and the ability to attain self-knowledge or direct perception of God.

Mental purity involves being pure in thought, word and action. In a pure mind there are no impurities, it sees purely and clearly. All impurities such as selfishness, greed, anger, jealousy, lust, hatred, resentment and other negative emotions are cleansed from the mind by the practice of yoga, meditation, constant awareness and surrender to God. Jesus said 'Blessed are the pure in heart, for they shall see God.' (Matthew 5:8)

1 Meditate and approach God with a pure heart.

Be open to His Will and His love, offering up all your desires and attachments to Him. Deep meditation cleanses the mind and body by removing tension and stress, allowing superconscious influences to flow into the mind.

In addition to meditation we can pray to God. Go into deep

meditation, then drop your meditation technique and enter the still silence within. During this silence commune with God by praying to Him sincerely to give you inner light and make you aware of the divine presence within you. The divine light which He radiates dispels the darkness of the heart. God who is love is seated in our hearts; by surrendering ourselves to His love in us, we become the embodiment of that love. Our life becomes pure and illumined with His power and love when we realize His presence within us, by constant remembrance and meditation.

The easiest way to purify the mind is to meditate and keep your thoughts on the pure truth within your heart. Prayer is the means to draw God's power, light and purity into us. Pray to Him, 'Beloved Lord make me pure in thought, word and action by revealing yourself in my heart.'

2 Discriminate and participate in regular *satsang*.

The coarser the object of pleasure, the more short-lived and unelevating is the pleasure arising out of it. Gambling, drinking, taking drugs, watching violent or pornographic videos for pleasure, are all examples of very unrefined pleasures. They do not satisfy our soul except for a short while, and they degrade the mind, making it impure and worldly. The excitement they cause is a waste of energy, and they cause suffering and pain, both mentally and physically.

The mind can also become impure by indiscriminately mixing with others who are selfishly self-centred, emotionally negative, weak-willed with bad habits, pleasure-seeking and greedy, lustful and hateful. It is like mixing clear, pure water with mud.

Satsang is a sanskrit word, meaning 'fellowship of truth'. In other words, keeping company or associating with those who are spiritually minded, who love God and live in truth. In such spiritual fellowship you may chant, pray, talk or meditate in silence. *Satsang* purifies one's consciousness. Jesus said: 'For where two or three are gathered together in my name, there I am in the midst of them.' (Matthew 18:20)

> *Environment is stronger than will-power. To mix with worldly people without absorbing at least some of their worldliness requires great spiritual strength ... whether one become a saint or sinner is to a great extent determined by the company he keeps.*
>
> Paramhansa Yogananda, from *The Essence of Self-Realization* by Sri Kriyananda

Environmental Cleanliness

It is also important to keep one's home and work environment clean and orderly. Our environment is a reflection of our mind. If our mind is impure, careless and disordered, then it will be reflected in our environment by being dirty, untidy and uncared for.

On a physical level dirt attracts germs, bacteria, insects and rodents. On an astral level dirt attracts disembodied lower entities.

Those that are heavily into tobacco, drugs and alcohol can also attract undesirable lower astral entities, which force their thought impressions on one's astral body and cling to one's aura. This may be one possible reason for a person's madness.

Cleanliness can also be thought of as order; our surroundings often reflect and affect us, so it is important to create a supportive environment. The clear, ordered mind can see positively in the most negative situations, and can help to clean or clear them up.

Bring order to your thoughts, feelings, behaviour and environment. 'Create in me a clean heart, O God and put a new and right spirit within me.' (Psalm 51: 10)

AFFIRMATION

I am now committed to a life of self-transformation and purification, to allow the radiance of the soul to unfold, and express itself clearly and purely.

I release all habits, attitudes and attachments which serve no useful purpose in my life.

I cleanse my mind of negative thoughts, feelings and emotions.

I live in harmony with nature's laws.

I live in the reality of God within me and around me. The reality of divine order is established in my mind and heart. I am a clear instrument for God's light.

SANTOSHA: CONTENTMENT

The Sanskrit word *santosha* has its root in the word *tush*, meaning 'to be pleased'. 'As a result of contentment one experiences supreme happiness.' (*The Yoga Sutras of Patanjali* 2:4)

> *Objective conditions are always neutral. It is how you react to them that makes them appear sad or happy.*
>
> *Work on yourself: on your reactions to outer circumstances. This is the essence of yoga: to neutralize the waves of reaction in the heart. Be happy inside. You will never be able to change things outwardly in such a way as to make them ever pleasing to you.*
>
> *Change yourself ... A good rule in life is to tell yourself simply, 'What comes of itself, let it come.'*
>
> Paramhansa Yogananda, from *The Essence of Self-Realization* by Sri Kriyananda

Contentment is a state of happiness and balance, accepting things as they are and being satisfied with what one has. To be content is also to have a true understanding and knowledge of one's own powers and limitations. Being content is accepting every moment as it is, without thinking that it should or could be different.

Live with awareness in the present moment, have no desire to know the nature of the next moment. Wishful thinking and anticipation often lead to disappointment, causing anxiety and tension, which drain one's energy.

Contentment is not a passive acceptance of one's physical and psychological circumstances and unnecessary sufferings and pain, or resignation to life. It does not mean that we should not make future plans, but rather that plans grow from our present reality, living in the present moment, rather than from dreaming and longing.

When we are content, we are happy. Happiness is a state of mind which is independent of circumstances, and does not depend upon any external condition at all. Our happiness should not be conditioned by what we have or do not have.

Happiness and unhappiness are states of the mind. The mind that is constantly changing and not contented cannot be satisfied permanently with anything. If a person is not content, their mind will restlessly wander, and they will find it impossible to concentrate and meditate.

Patanjali says in the first chapter of his *Sutras*: 'Yoga (union) is the stilling of the movement of thought.'

When all conflict and confusion in the mind are resolved, there is no thought. The mind becomes still, and from this stillness of thought arises contentment, which brings a continuous flow of happiness and inner peace.

Contentment is closely related to equanimity (*samata*), which means being equal-minded, calmness of mind, freedom from attachment and aversion.

There are references to both contentment and equanimity in the *Bhagavad Gita*. Krishna says:

> *That person of action is free from karma who accepts with contentment whatever comes to them, who is free from jealousy, and has transcended all dualities of life, and who is balanced in success and failure.*
>
> Bhagavad Gita, 4:22

> *Those whose minds are established in equanimity [equal-mindedness] are free from the relativities of existence (birth and death, pleasure and pain), even in this world.*
>
> *They are flawless like the Supreme Reality. With even mind they are already situated in pure consciousness ...*
>
> *Being fixed in deep communion with the eternal Supreme Truth, with unwavering discrimination and free from delusion, they never became falsely elated by pleasant experiences or depressed by bad.*
>
> Bhagavad Gita 5:19-20

THE PRACTICE OF *SANTOSHA*

1 Do not allow desires to control your thoughts.

If you allow desires to control your thoughts, your mind will become restless and discontent. Watch your thoughts carefully and try to understand from where desire arises. The process of desire is as follows:

1 The eyes look at a beautiful object.
2 The mind comes in, registers it and takes a mental picture.
3 Now that the mind is coloured by that picture, it keeps recurring. The imagination (*vikalpa*) and memory (*smriti*) provide motivation.
4 This creates a desire, a craving. The craving arises even when the object is not present. The mind, unfulfilled and discontent, continually thinks of the object.

If the object you desire is not here, then be content in this moment.

Tell your mind, 'The object you desire is not here, be content with what you have here and now.'

Ask yourself, 'Is it really necessary to have this object?' Hunger, thirst and even the need to love and be loved are all part of life, but in none of these is there an agitated craving. Ask yourself, 'What is it that craves, what is craving?'

Three things are constantly working within us, which cause discontent and restlessness in the mind: desire and craving; dislike or hate; and fear.

Fear is created as follows:
1 From ignorance (*avidya*) of what is truth, ego-sense (*asmita*) arises.
2 Ego-sense is 'I'. The 'I' creates division: 'I like this' leads to approval (*raga*); 'I don't like this' leads to dissapproval (*dvesha*).
3 Imagination (*vikalpa*) and memory (*smriti*) influence our approval or disapproval.
4 From the ego's division of 'I like' and 'I don't like', fear is created. Fear results from non-acceptance of what is. If we are content we accept what is, there is no fear.

The mind is made restless by ignorance [lack of self awareness], egoism, attraction and repulsion, likes and dislikes, clinging to life and fear of death.

The Yoga Sutras of Patanjali, 2:3

Let life flow on, accept it. Do not allow your consciousness to be coloured by approval and disapproval.

2 Live in the present moment.

Be content and happy with what you have. Do not hanker after things. True happiness and freedom are inner states which you attain when you are in tune with God, who dwells within you.

3 Be still within.

Restless thoughts are caused by desires and attachment, which in turn create discontent, anger, jealousy, hate and fear.

The mind is like a lake – its natural state is to be calm and crystal clear. To the lake itself there is no motion, no change, no waves, ripples or currents, but the thoughts, ideas and images (*vrittis*), those innumerable waves with which one identifies oneself, agitate the mind into restless activity, obscuring its true nature.

These thoughts can either arise from the bottom of the lake (memories), or from our sense perceptions, and imagination. When the ripples of the mind are stilled and it becomes crystal clear, then we can see the reflection of the infinite spirit.

To bring peace and stillness to the mind, first withdraw it from its attraction to different objects. Then make the mind one-pointed by concentrating on that reality of truth which is God. The mind absorbed in the object of meditation becomes silenced; this silence and stillness brings contentment, joy, calmness, peace and higher awareness.

4 Surrender your will to God's Will.

Surrender means inner contentment and peace. Surrender your will to God's Will and be content with all situations and circumstances in which God places you. 'Teach me to do Thy Will, for thou art my God.' (Psalm 143:10)

5 Be non-attached.

Contentment is being able to receive whatever comes naturally for satisfying the needs of our body, mind and soul. Make good use of those things which come to you in a useful and purposeful way, without becoming attached to them.

When one has contentment then austerity follows naturally as a simple way of living.

6 Keep your life simple.

Make this your maxim: 'Simple living, high thinking.' Follow the middle path, be balanced and moderate in all things.

7 Learn from inner experience.

The experiences that come to us are not as important as what we learn and become through them.

AFFIRMATION

In the still depths of the soul, I am undisturbed by the surface waves of experiences. God's spirit resides within me, content and peaceful.

Whatever comes of itself I expect, and I remain calmly centred within. Within me lies the source of true joy and peace.
I perform all action, while inwardly united with the joy of the soul.
I live life now in the present moment.
I remain open and receptive to positive changes in my life.

The wisdom of God is present and active within me. From this wisdom I gain awareness of the Self, insight, understanding and harmony of the body, mind and soul, which are necessary to bring contentment and peace into my life.

TAPAS: AUSTERITY

'Austerity or self-discipline destroys all impurities of the mind. From this arises perfection of the body, mind and senses.' (*The Yoga Sutras of Patanjali*, 2:34)

Tapas literally means 'heat (inner fire)'. When there is heat, there is also energy. *Tapas* is energy that is concentrated or focused with conscious will-power on a specific point, so that it releases power and sets it in motion. This is likened to concentrating the sun's rays through a magnifying glass over a piece of paper. The heat is concentrated and intensified into a single fine ray of light, which produces a powerful energy to burn the paper.

The practice of *tapas* enables one to strengthen a firm resolve and develop a strong will-power to overcome the egoistic nature of the mind. *Tapas* helps one to control and direct the power of the mind and body for higher spiritual aims and purposes.

The practice of austerity has an ancient history in both the West and the East. During the period of St Anthony (born about 251 AD and thought to be the founder of monasticism), the early Christian monks (the 'desert fathers') lived in desert caves, seeking God through a life of austerity, asceticism, meditation and prayer. The ascetic practices of the Western monks at that time were very similar to those practised in the East by Indian monks or yogis (about 300 AD, about the time when Patanjali's school of yoga was being taught).

It is important to understand that *tapas* is not an end in itself. Tapas should be practised with intelligence and discrimination. To torture the body and mind, and make the senses dull and unresponsive, is *not* the object. *Tapas* practised in the true spirit of yoga is not penance (an act performed through feelings of regret that one has committed a sin). To whip one's own body or lie on a bed of nails is *not* part of the yogic attitude towards life; this is denying life in a negative way. The ascetic pursues pain to avoid pleasure and the worldly person seeks pleasure to avoid pain. In both, pain is inseparable from pleasure. When we pursue pleasure or pain, we deny ourselves freedom, peace and joy in life. We have to find a balance between indulgence and abstinence. Through yoga disciplines we can train our bodies and senses to be useful instruments of selfless service to others. In this way our minds become purified and we can make a positive contribution to life.

When we have control over the mind and its modifications, and the senses are naturally and spontaneously regulated, the body and mind become clear channels for the soul within to express itself naturally and clearly. The object then of *tapas* is to train the body, mind and senses to become steady and balanced so that they work naturally, spontaneously and selflessly for the soul to express itself purely.

The following verses from the *Bhagavad Gita* enlighten us on the practice of austerity.

> *The yogi is thought to be superior to the ascetics, and even greater than those following the path of knowledge [Jnana Yoga] or to those who perform action [Karma Yoga].*
>
> 6:46

> *Even among all yogis, that man or woman who is absorbed in Me, with their soul completely immersed in Me, is considered by Me to be the superior yogi.*
>
> 6:47

The word 'yogi' refers to one who practises meditation on the self within, who is self-disciplined, free from self-centred attachments, desires and egotism, and who is contented and equal-minded.

Krishna informs us that we have to find a balance between indulgence and abstinence.

> *Arjuna, those who eat too much or eat too little, who sleep too much or too little do not find success in yoga.*
>
> 6:16

> *Those that are regulated and balanced in eating, sleeping, work and recreation find an end to sorrow through yoga.*
>
> 6:17

Later, in chapter 17, Krishna informs us that there are certain people who torment their minds and torture their bodies by practising too severe asceticism. In fact, it is the subtle force of their attachment to sense pleasure that moves them to such severity!

> *Those people who practise severe austerities not authorized by the scriptures, motivated by hypocrisy and egoism, impelled by lust, and attachment, unintelligently and senselessly torture their bodies and offend Me, the Soul dwelling within.*
>
> 17:5-6

> *Those ostentatious austerities which are practised with the object of gaining respect, honour and admiration are said to be rajasic (in the mode of passion), unstable and transitory.*
>
> *Austerities which are practised foolishly, with self-torture, or for injuring others, are said to be tamasic (in the mode of ignorance).*
>
> 17:18-19

The Practice of *Tapas*

In chapter 17 of the *Bhagavad Gita*, Krishna outlines three types of austerity: for the *body*, *speech* and *mind*. He says in verse 17:

> *This threefold austerity performed by people who are persevering with great faith, and who desire no reward for their actions, is sattvic (in the mode of goodness).*

1 Austerity of the body

> *Be serviceful to God, to the good, the wise and the gurus. Purity [cleanliness], honesty, simplicity, continence and non-violence are considered the austerity of the body.*
>
> 17:14

2 Austerity of speech

> *To speak words that are truthful, kind and helpful, that cause no resentment, and to regularly study the scriptures, are called the austerity of speech.*
>
> 17:15

3 Austerity of the mind

Calmness, kindness, silence, self-control and purity of thought are called austerity of mind.
17:16

To be serviceful to God, to the good, the wise and the gurus, means to give respect, and render service unconditionally. We are reflected lights of God, and our origin is in God. To always remember God with our awareness in Him and being surrendered in God is the greatest service we can give to God. The universe is manifested to serve God's Will and we are here to serve God's Will, and to serve others in God.

We are also here to co-operate with evolutionary forces and God's representatives, who are God-conscious and surrendered to His Will.

By the practice of these threefold austerities all afflictions and impurities of the mind and the body are removed, making them strong and healthy.

The attitude for practising austerity is with perfect inner contentment. When one has contentment then austerity follows naturally as a simple way of living. Our desires, wants and needs are reduced with contentment, resulting in greater sensitivity.

Remember, it is not by beating or starving the body, by tormenting the mind or by breaking the senses that we attain self-realization. We have to give the physical body what it needs to function as a healthy, sensitive organism, and deny it those things which are unnecessary. Good bodily and mental health is essential to spiritual life. Our mind and body can serve God and others when they are in good health, with energy and vitality.

Of the threefold austerities, mental austerity is the most powerful. If the mind is mastered then body and speech will come under its control more easily.

AFFIRMATION

I am made in the image and likeness of God, my body is the temple of spirit, it is a perfect expression of radiant health that God created it to be. I respect my body by keeping it clean and living by natural laws relative to exercise, diet, rest and relaxation.

I am attuned to the truth of my being – my true spiritual nature – by remembering and giving service to God first in my mind and heart. I also respect and listen to the wisdom of the enlightened sages, saints and gurus. I serve the cause of evolution by serving God and the wise.

I choose to live God-consciously with soul-awareness, mental clarity, radiant physical health, emotional maturity, and a simple, balanced moderate lifestyle that supports my spiritual growth and relationship with God.

I express my thoughts and feelings in positive words that are truthful, helpful and kind to others. I release all limiting feelings, behaviours and attitudes that keep me from recognizing and experiencing my true spiritual nature. I give expression to inner joy and calmness. I open myself to infinite good so that the blessings of life flow through me to others.

SVADHYAYA: SELF-STUDY

'By study of the scriptures and oneself one is united with that loved aspect of divinity.' (*The Yoga Sutras of Patanjali*, 2:44)

Sva means 'self (one's own)'. *Adhyaya* means 'study'. So *svadyhaya* literally means 'self-study'.

Patanjali also says:

> Austerity, study of the scriptures and one's own awareness of situations from moment to moment, surrender of self-consciousness [egotism] and dedicating the fruits of one's actions to God, is the path of Kriya Yoga [active yoga or working towards God].
>
> The Yoga Sutras of Patanjali, 2:1

Svadhyaya can also mean the study of scriptural texts and the silent recitation of mantras to oneself. The mental repetition of mantras in this way is called *japa*. Both the study of scriptural texts and mantra *japa* are to be practised in a meditative and concentrated state of absorbed awareness.

The basis for self-study is concentrated within all the *yamas* and *niyamas*. These confront our involvement with all of life around us and then slowly centre in a study of our inner self.

When one has become established in the first three *niyamas* – *saucha*, *santosha* and *tapas* – then one is ready for self-study, self-introspection or self-awareness. In self-study one learns not by gaining intellectual or material knowledge but by standing back to observe, and to study the studier. It is by observing with awareness our own thoughts, feelings, behaviour, desires, motives and attitudes that we can see the delusions, false attachments and ignorance that prevent us from realizing our true soul-nature.

The practice of *svadhaya* encourages spiritual awakening in us, so that we can realize our divine nature and the reality of God.

At the deepest level of our inner being we are pure consciousness, made in the image and likeness of God. If we do not know this, it is because of self-forgetfulness and ignorance due to identification with the mind and the objects of the senses. All our problems in life ultimately stem from our *separation* from the source of our divinity, which is God.

Most people live primarily for themselves and their families; their vision seldom reaches higher than that. Society (politicians, teachers, parents, the advertising media) teaches and conditions us to look outside of ourselves for happiness and fulfilment. But the great Masters tell us differently. Jesus said: 'The Kingdom of God is within you.' (Luke 17:21) He also said: 'But seek ye first the Kingdom of God, and His righteousness; and all these things shall be added unto you.' (Matthew 6:33) And in the *Bhagavad Gita*, Lord Krishna says:

> To those who meditate on Me as their very own, ever united to Me by incessant worship, I provide their deficiencies and make permanent their gain.
>
> 9:22

The Kingdom of God, which is infinite intelligence, wisdom, love, joy and inner peace is within each one of us. These qualities are within us because they are in God, and we are made in the image and likeness of God. Each one of us is an expression of God-consciousness, using God-faculties and expressing God-qualities. But until we awaken to this fact of life, and experience the presence of God within, knowing that we have free will to choose and can direct our mind, control our emotions, senses and body, we continue to be in an unaware, conditioned state of sleep. In this state of somnolence or ignorance the Spirit of God dwelling in us cannot express itself in all its light and glory; the soul's potential is in effect thwarted. In this conditioned state of sleep we are delayed in attaining our perfect and complete experience of superconscious union with God.

The Practice of Svadhaya

When you awaken to your true nature within, you will grow into the light, which will remove all darkness and unknowing from your mind and consciousness. With soul-awareness in God you will be able to control your own destiny, living a life guided by the divine spirit within, governed by truth.

God cannot be completely understood or realized through the intellectual process. Self-study must begin with awareness and an understanding of the mind's movements, the study of the nature of thought and the thinking process. What is thought? How does it arise? What are its functions and limitations? Self-study is not an intellectual process, but simply a perceptive *awareness* of the movements of the mind, which arises through our distraction from moment to moment. When we recognize our distraction or lack of awareness we can discover our true identity and reality *as it is*. All that is needed is simple attention to what is happening in us and around us in each moment. Whether we are breathing, meditating, chanting, cooking, eating, working or studying, if we do it with attentive awareness and alertness, each moment will be a freeing experience, in which we will see and understand something new.

Life requires of us to be constantly in clear awareness, with a quiet, meditative mind which is full of energy, love and compassion, a mind which is free from past conditioning, reactive behaviour patterns, subconscious motivations, habitual ego-centred behaviour, sense-urges negative emotions and negative attitudes. In the quiet, aware and alert mind there is true freedom from tension, conflict and sorrow. There is a direct perception of life without distortion.

Without attentive awareness and alertness, our consciousness becomes clouded, we become sleepy and our senses lose their sensitivity and become dull. When our attention and sensitivity are sharpened and heightened with awareness, our perception becomes clear. In this state of observation we are able to perceive and recognize those limiting conditions within our minds that prevent us from fulfilling our true potential and destiny in life. With inner awareness we can understand why the mind is distracted and inattentive. In unbroken, clear awareness we can decondition and dehypnotize the mind of its subconscious motivations, ignorance, addictions and bad habits.

Self-awareness begins with you here and now in this moment, in every moment of your life. When you live every moment in awareness, you will experience the Eternal as a living reality. The average person only uses a tiny fraction of awareness in his or her everyday living. We go from one day to the next throughout life in a state of distraction, unawareness and restlessness. Half-heartedly we go through all the activities of the day in a somnolent state of awareness, and the beauty of life escapes us. In this conditioned state of mind we are mostly attentive to our subconscious motives, and therefore our perception is distorted. We are not even aware or mindful when eating our meals, cleaning our teeth or listening when someone is talking to us. Perhaps you go to the bathroom or kitchen and leave it untidy or dirty, burn the toast, leave water running from a tap, or forget to switch a light or heater off before you go out. They may be small activities in your life, but the way to self-realization lies through the sensitivity, awareness, care and attention to all that we do in thought, word and action, no matter how small it may seem. We need to live each moment of our life completely, carefully observing all the details with constant awareness and attention. It is only when we perceive clearly and live truly in accord with life's processes that the reality of God is glorified through us.

It does not matter how long you have been sitting in the dark; when light is brought in, the darkness disappears. It is our responsibility to awake in the light, to consciously know our true nature and reality as the self. With knowledge, understanding and mastery of our mind, body and senses, we can direct our lives intelligently and superconsciously, expressing ourselves in a balanced and fulfilling way on all levels of our being.

Self-knowledge or self-awareness is not a goal to seek. The Self *is* knowledge. Self-awareness cannot be divided from awareness, which is the Self.

Self-knowledge is the awareness of the immortal reality within us, which sets us free from the bondage of ignorance, the cause of all our sorrows. This knowledge and awareness, which is the Self, is here and now, always. It has never ceased to be, and so is not a goal that we have to search for.

There is no mystery to it. All we need to do is remove the obstacles, dispelling the ignorance that obscures the Self *as* knowledge. The sun is always shining, but when it is obscured by dark clouds we do not see it. When the clouds disperse then the sun becomes visible and the light shines.

Patanjali, in his *Yoga Sutras* instructs us how to remove ignorance effectively: 'The practice of uninterrupted awareness and discrimination between what is real and what is unreal, removes obstacles [ignorance].' (2:26)

The intelligent practice of the first seven of the eight limbs of yoga with uninterrupted awareness, gives us the basic methods in removing ignorance. If we are to remain in the light of Self-knowledge, then we need to be vigilant, constantly awake, alert and aware in every moment. This is no part-time exercise; the practice of yoga once taken up, involves your entire life. This total approach to life reveals your commitment to awakening in God-consciousness. If we are unmotivated, uncommitted and practising only half-heartedly we cannot expect complete success and fulfilment in this incarnation. We must sincerely want to awaken from our ignorance, and become surrendered and actively involved in our own spiritual unfoldment.

Yoga is basically the removal of obstacles and obstructions from the mind and body, so that the inner joy and light of the Self that is already here (but is not shining because of obstructions, ignorance and misunderstanding) can shine in perfect Self-awareness.

In his *Sutras* (1:30) Patanjali lists nine main obstacles that distract the mind.

Disease (*Vyadhi*)

'A healthy body is the guest chamber of the soul; a sick one its prison.' (Francis Bacon, *Augmentis Scientarum: Valetudo*)

Disease means loss of ease, balance and harmony, it means there is tension within. If the body and mind are in balance, disease will not occur. We need a healthy mind in a healthy body that we may have sufficient time and opportunity to evolve into the realization of the immortal nature of the Self and fulfil the real purpose of human experience and all the possibilities of life.

The mind and body are instruments of the Self; if either of them become dis-eased or imbalanced, the Self will not be able to express through them as it would in a healthy mind and physiology.

The more pure and refined the mind and physiology are, the easier it is for superconscious soul-influences to express through them.

Our spiritual progress can be restricted by a dis-eased mind and body. For example, if you are ill, and your body is in pain and feeling weak, it is difficult to sit calmly in meditation. Your mind is distracted by the physical pain and discomfort. You are unable to concentrate or become focused clearly in meditation.

The mind exerts the deepest influence on the body. With constant awareness and intentional discipline we can consciously create a healthy mind and physiology, maintaining a balance.

The following are the prerequisites of natural immunity to disease.

1 Live in harmony with natural laws.

2 Maintain a clean, healthy bloodstream.

This comes from pure nutrition, pure water, pure air, good digestion and efficient elimination.

3 Take regular daily exercise.

This strengthens, stretches, gives stamina, and tones the internal body organs and systems.

4 Breathe properly.

5 Get sufficient rest, sleep and relaxation.

6 Meditate.

7 Maintain a positive, cheerful, mental outlook on life in all circumstances.

Do the best you can in any circumstance and leave the rest to God.

Mental Laziness, Procrastination (*Styana*).

To overcome this obstacle:

1 Establish your priorities.

Give conscious attention to important matters such as meditation.

2 Determine your current life priority and direction, then live with intention.

3 Identify those habits that are preventing you from giving attention to important priorities, purpose and direction in life.

4 Be more purposeful, willing and enthusiastic.

Develop an interest in all that you do.

5 Be disciplined with interest and enthusiasm in your daily routines and spiritual practices.

Develop a keen interest in pursuits that will help you attain self-mastery.

6 Develop the power of concentration and think clearly.

A person with a distracted, restless mind cannot achieve anything. Tremendous power flows into us when we concentrate and are absorbed in God.

7 Do not put off what you can do now.

If you procrastinate you will never achieve your aims in life. Change your mental attitude and become motivated and willing to make the right effort now. Never accept failure – if you do so, you will become a failure and deny the power of God within you. Be determined and resolve never to cease trying to do your best. If you are making a continuous effort now, you cannot fail.

8 Make good use of your time, for every moment is precious.

Do not waste your time and restrict your spiritual unfoldment by being idle. Remember, life is very short, there is no time to lose in awakening in God-consciousness. Be clearly aware of your true purpose for being here and make the most of every available opportunity.

9 Practise introspection.

Keep a mental diary of what you are doing and thinking throughout the day. Constructively analyse your bad habits and find the cause. Why is it that you are lazy or are procrastinating? How did you acquire the negative traits? Be discriminating and recognize your weaknesses, then remove them from your consciousness. Resolve to make a positive change in your life and affirm aloud with firm conviction:

> *Today I make a commitment to move willingly in a purposeful direction to fulfil my spiritual aim in life – to develop a closer, deeper relationship with God.*
>
> *I make wise use of my time, energy and talents. I am positive! I am energetic! I am enthusiastic!*
>
> *I consciously and attentively practise necessary disciplines and practices in my daily routine, to attain self-mastery and realize my unity with God.*

10 Create more energy.

Yogananda said, 'Will power directs energy, and energy in turn acts upon matter. Matter, indeed, *is* energy. The stronger the will, the greater the force of energy.' (from *The Essence of Self-Realisation* by Sri Kriyananda) Energy is an important key to spiritual life. All matter, including human beings, is in reality energy. Energy is infinite, it has no limitation and we can tap into it and draw from this universal energy as much as we want to.

Yogananda also said, 'Joy and energy go hand in hand.' If you have high energy you cannot be sad, and if you are joyful, you have energy. Look at people who are depressed. Everyone who is depressed has low energy, and one of the most difficult things psychologists have to do with people who are depressed is to get them to do something about it. There is no energy flowing in a depressed person, but people who are joyful are full of energy.

Unwillingness, boredom, moodiness and fear of failure are all mental energy blocks that we should work to overcome.

When we bring our will in tune with God's Will we become unlimited; in this way will-power makes us divine.

The greatest use for our will-power is to use it to meditate. God wants us to discover our divine will and use it to find and commune with Him.

Doubt (*Samshaya*)

Doubts are our worst enemy. When the mind is in doubt it becomes undecided, uncertain, and even disbelieving. The mind becomes torn between different possibilities, jumping from one to the other, becoming more and more confused.

If you have doubts about the existence of God, the scriptural texts, the tradition of your guru and his teachings, or your own inner reality and your purpose in life, then clear your confusion and resolve your doubts by developing faith and confidence. Knowledge removes doubt.

Depending on one's attitude, doubt can be positive and expand our awareness, or negative and destructive, resulting in a depressive mood. When you are in doubt ask yourself, 'Am I in doubt so that I will not have to act, enabling me to escape from responsibility and commitment or am I in doubt because I intuitively feel that something is not quite right?' Positive doubt that stimulates genuine enquiry can expand our awareness. Negative doubt created through restlessness and impatience arising from the ego decreases our awareness.

Meditate deeply, so that you develop your power of intuition. After meditation remain calmly seated in the silence and pray to God for faith, strength and guidance to overcome your doubts. When your emotions are settled and your mind is free from restlessness and confusion, then you will be able to clear your doubts.

Carelessness, Negligence (*Pramada*)

Negligence is failing to be consciously attentive, and being uninterested in your spiritual practices and disciplines. Cultivate a sincere interest in your spiritual unfoldment. Be intentional in your spiritual practices and disciplines. Resolve now to be committed to living perfectly with clear understanding and resolve to express God's will.

If you are aware of higher realities but are still continuing to act from conditioned and habitual ways, your spiritual growth will be restricted and limited.

Sloth, Lethargy (*Alasya*)

Laziness is failure to progress spiritually due to lack of perseverance, willingness and enthusiasm, with an extreme lack of energy or vitality (or in the state of *tamas*).

There is a mammal called a sloth, which is of a sluggish, slow-moving nature, which inhabits tropical parts of Central and South America. There are also human beings who are sluggish, physically and mentally. Disinclined to exertion, they move slowly and pass their time in idleness. This is the tamasic state that Lord Krishna mentions in the *Bhagavad Gita*, chapter 17.

Paramhansa Yogananda once said, 'I can forgive the physically lazy person, but not the mentally lazy person.' What he meant by this was that sometimes the physically lazy person can be excused if the laziness is due to ill health, but mental laziness is inexcusable for those who choose to be unwilling, unmotivated, with no self-effort.

To overcome inertia and laziness one needs to purify and energize the physical body and mind to rise to the sattvic state. The mind and body are inseparable – if the body is not nourished with a healthy balanced vegetarian diet, the mind is affected. A diet of heavy food, meat, alcohol, drugs and smoking causes inertia and heaviness in the body and mental field.

Too much eating and sleeping for long hours with little or no exercise is also a cause of lethargy.

Attachment to Sense-Pleasure (*Avirati*)

Our desire or need for someone or something apart from God creates a sense of separation from Him, or makes us believe that we could be satisfied without His power and presence. The more we desire the more we become attached. Attachment deepens our desires. Attachment to sense-pleasures prevents us from concentrating on our spiritual reality. When our mind is distracted by strong ego-needs and outer sources of sense stimulation, we lose our self-awareness, and become mentally restless, confused and emotionally unsettled.

We need to regulate our sense-pleasures and bring them into balance. This requires careful discrimination and complete, clear understanding of our emotions, so that we can withdraw energy from them and dissolve them.

Distorted Vision, Philosophical Confusion (*Bhranti Darshana*)

Due to false perception, ignorance, ego-sense and lack of understanding we may totally reject philosophical truths that great saints and sages or yogic scriptures have taught us.

If we are mentally confused and misunderstand the nature of God and the universe, we can improve our understanding by developing faith in God and the great Masters. Study the teachings of the great respected Masters: Jesus Christ, Lord Krishna, Patanjali and Paramhansa Yogananda are a few, but there are also others. Read and study the great classic scriptures: the New Testament, the *Bhagavad Gita*, *The Yoga Sutras of Patanjali*, and the *Upanishads*. Read also Paramhansa Yogananda's *Autobiography of A Yogi*. This book has inspired thousands of truth-seekers.

Meditate deeply with a clear calm mind and pray to God:

Dear Lord, make me pure in thought, word and deed by revealing yourself in my heart. Clear all confusion and error from my mind and awaken in me Thy truth – om, peace, amen.

Failure to Gain a Firm Ground in Yoga (*Alabdha Bhumikatva*)

We may fail to make progress to the higher stages of yoga, even though we have been observing the proper practices.

Patanjali says:

> *That practice becomes firm in ground only when spontaneous awareness continues with consistent efforts without interruption for a long time.*
>
> The Yoga Sutras of Patanjali, 1:14

We need to be consistent and constant in our efforts towards self-realization, with clear, spontaneous awareness, without distraction, sincerely and earnestly devoted to practising the presence of God. (In all that you do, remain centred in the awareness of God.)

True spirituality consists in our living in this world and giving service to all beings, while all the time being consciously aware of the divine self within and around us.

Instability, Unsteadiness of Mind (*Anasthitatva*)

The obstacle here, is that one may gain a higher stage of yoga, but fall from it, or be unable to maintain oneself there due to the unsteadiness and inattention of the mind.

Patanjali (*Yoga Sutras* 1:31) identifies four secondary obstacles as symptoms of a distracted mind.

Pain, Grief and Sorrow (*Duhkha*)

When you experience pain, unhappiness or sorrow, the mind is attracted to it. The mind is distracted from that which is beyond pain – the Self. One is unable to meditate when the mind is distracted by painful memories, emotional hurts and painful desires.

There are three kinds of pain:
- *adhyatmika* – within oneself (physical, mental and emotional)
- *adhibhautika* – caused by other beings (including wild animals and insects)
- *adhidaivika* – caused by natural forces (sound, air, fire, water, earth and planetary forces)

Eliminate pain by examining it. Look at it and become aware of it. Who or what is experiencing pain? How does that 'I' experience arise? Why does it not arise in sleep? Have you ever wondered why the 'I' experience does not exist in sleep? Why the sleeping person does not say 'I sleep?' Why is it that you do not feel pain when you are asleep? In sleep there is a division of the 'I' from the experience.

Psychological Despair

Again, meditation is disturbed by the mind being distracted by negative moods, frustration, negative thoughts, anxiety and ill-will.

Moods are the result of low or negative energy. Change the energy level and its direction and you will develop a positive state of mind. Paramhansa Yogananda said once to a certain disciple, who was inclined to be moody:

> *If you want to be sad ... no one in the world can make you happy. But if you make up your mind to be happy, no one and nothing on earth can take that happiness from you.*
>
> from *The Essence of Self-Realisation* by Sri Kriyananda

You can overcome a mood with the following practice.

1 **Exercise vigorously.**

2 **Concentrate your attention at the point between the eyebrows (the spiritual eye) for five minutes and will yourself into the superconscious.**

3 **Seek cheerful company.**

4 **Affirm with a cheerful attitude:**

I am not my moods, and I am not subject to the moods of others. I am ruler in my kingdom of thoughts and feelings! I am positive! The joy of God fills my mind with cheerful thoughts.

5 **Be busy in constructive and useful activity.**

6 **Be devoted selflessly to helping others.**

7 **Chant or sing from the heart joyously.**

Unsteadiness of the Body During Meditation

When the body is restless, twitching and itching, it is difficult to focus your attention in meditation.

By the regular practice of yoga postures (*asanas*), one can make the body sit comfortably and steady. In meditation you must be able to hold your seated posture absolutely steady and still with no movement. If the body is not still the mind becomes distracted.

Irregular Inhalation and Exhalation

Uneven inhalation and exhalation is caused by fluctuations of the mind and emotional instability.

If you are attentive to your breathing, you will be aware of the degree of distractedness of the mind. The less distracted it is, the calmer the breathing is; the more distracted, the more restless and irregular the breathing is.

If you want to know what total absorption of the mind is, exhale and suspend your breathing. It is the breath (or the movement of the *prana*) that enables your mind to think. If you suspend the breath, the mind loses its fuel and becomes quiet and still. This is what happens in deep meditation, where there is total absorption of the mind.

Japa

Mental or silent repetition (*japa*) of that aspect of divinity chosen for worship is considered by saints and sages to be better than verbal repetition. With mental repetition, the mind is fixed in the Name, whereas oral repetition does not effectively stop the mind from wandering, unless the mind is absorbed in the sound of the Name.

If your mind wanders while chanting mentally or aloud, your love and devotion for God cannot be very great. If you really love God above everything else, His Name will give you joy instantly. Where one's love is, there one's mind is. Any object or person that you love with all your heart gives you great joy, just by the thought of it.

By chanting God's Name, ever remembering Him, by keeping your mind in tune with God, in course of time you will develop a steady and unbroken consciousness of God.

Japa means 'repetition'. *Japa* is the repetition of a mantra; this Sanskrit word comes from *manas* ('mind'), and *tri* ('to cross over'). So, a mantra is a spiritual, mystical formula or holy Name which is inherently connected with the reality it represents. Mantra liberates the consciousness, it helps us to cross over the sea of the uncontrolled and conditioned mind.

The practice of *japa* yoga can help us to maintain a continuous remembrance of God. *Japa* is thinking of God constantly, to the exclusion of everything else. Repetition of the Names of God or mantra with sincerity, faith, one-pointed concentration and devotion keeps away all other thoughts. It is the power that we infuse into the word that produces the effect. When we repeat the Name of God with love and devotion, it sets up a vibration that keeps our mind and senses harmonized with the divine within us.

With constant practice of *japa* one can transcend the mind and realize one's identity with God.

There are four main categories of *japa*.

- ***vaikhari japa.*** The mantra is spoken or chanted aloud. This form of *japa* is particularly good for those people who are negatively emotional, dull, moody or of a restless nature. When *vaikhari japa* is practised alone or in a group of people the atmosphere becomes powerfully charged with positive vibrations of peace, joy and energy.

  When chanting aloud, chant with love and devotion. Concentrate at the spiritual eye (the point between the eyebrows), drawing God's energy and joy to you. Open your heart and listen attentively to the sound of the mantra that you are chanting. Sound is easy for the mind to concentrate upon. When the mind is absorbed in the mantric vibration of sound, we rise higher into a state of superconsciousness. It is then that the chanter, the chant and the process of chanting become one.

- ***upansu japa.*** The mantra is *whispered*. Only the one who is chanting the mantra can hear it. This form of *japa* is useful for those people who are practising many hours of *japa* throughout the day. It is also good for those who are practising *japa* with a special mantra for a specific purpose. Practise this for three months before you begin *manasika japa*.

- ***manasika japa.*** The mantra is repeated *mentally*. There is no movement of the lips. This is the most subtle *japa* and can be difficult for beginners in the practice of mantra yoga. The mind can easily be sidetracked and wander away from the practice to other thoughts. During this practice, if you are not vigilant and attentive, sleep may overpower you. This higher practice is for those who are able to concentrate with a steady mind.

  When practising mental *japa*, or any other form, the mantra should not be repeated mechanically or in a hurry without love, devotion and faith. When mental *japa* is repeated with deep concentration, attention and awareness, it prepares the mind for meditation on God.

- ***likhita japa.*** The mantra is *written*, while being simultaneously repeated mentally. It is written down on paper hundreds or thousands of times in lines, shapes or forms (such as the shape of a lotus flower or a mandala). It is best to keep a notebook specifically for this purpose; it can be kept near your bed or the shrine where you meditate.

When you write the mantra use red ink, as this will help to reinforce the mantra in your mind. Blue and green ink can also be used. Write the letters of the mantra as small as possible, carefully creating a beautiful design. Practise with concentration and devotion. It is also good to concentrate on the meaning of the mantra so that it predominates over other thoughts.

Ajapa Japa

Ajapa japa is the spontaneous and automatic repetition of the mantra or Name of God without conscious effort. It is a combination of *pranayama* (see chapter 5) and *meditation* (see chapter 8). In *ajapa japa* it is important to be consciously attentive and aware of one's own natural breath and its movement or flow through the body (*ujjayi pranayama*).

In the practice of *ajapa japa* the awareness of the natural flow of the breath or *ujjayi pranayama* is integrated with the mantra *soham* ('I am He'). *Soham* is a Vedantic mantra found in the *Isa-Upanishad*. The word *hamsa* meaning 'swan' is a symbol of supreme Reality and has the mantra *so'ham aham sah* ('I am He, He is me') within it. *Aham* ('I') and *sah* ('He') mean, 'I am one with Spirit'. The letters *s* and *h* in the mantra *soham* are consonants, which represent the names and forms in this universe, their fleeting and temporary nature. If we remove the *s* and *h*, we are left with *oam* or *om*, the only true reality, the soul of your breath.

In this practice the breath and mantra become one as they are rotated up and down the spine, between the base chakra (*muladhara*) and the spiritual eye (*ajna chakra*).

There are other variations of the mantra used by different schools of yoga, such as *hang-sah*. *Hang* represents *aham*, the personal pronoun 'I', and *sah* represents the Cosmic Self. In practising this mantric *kriya* the ego and the Self become one.

The mantra *hong sau* (pronounced '*hong saw*') also means 'I am He' (I am one with Spirit), but whereas *soham* relates to concentration on the currents of energy in the spine, *hong sau* is a mantra for developing deep concentration on the breath with the attention at the spiritual eye (*ajna chakra*).

> *If you want to be a Master in this lifetime, Yogananda told a disciple, then, along with your other meditation practices, practise* hong sau *at least two hours a day.*
>
> *As a boy, I use to practise* hong sau *sometimes for seven hours at a time, until I entered the breathless state of ecstasy.*
>
> from *The Essence of Self-Realization* by Sri Kriyananda

If we can repeat this mantra constantly until it becomes integrated within our consciousness and is always present in the mind, we will realize our oneness with God.

Every day, the breath rises naturally, making the sound *so*, and falls, making the sound *hum*, 21,600 times. Very few people are aware of their breath throughout the day. The following practice of *ajapa japa* develops awareness and concentration, and is the basis for Kriya Yoga. One achieves *pratyahara* (sense-withdrawal) by mastering the practice of this technique.

1. Sit in a meditational posture and close the eyes. Keep the body still and relaxed, with the eyes focused at the spiritual eye (*ajna chakra*).
2. Begin to observe, with awareness, the natural flow of the breath for a few minutes.
3. Now bring your awareness to the psychic passage within the spine and feel the rising breath from the base of the spine (*muladhara chakra*) to the base of the brain (medulla oblongata). With this inhalation mentally synchronize and listen to the mantric sound *so*. Then, exhaling down the spine from the medulla oblongata to the *muladhara chakra*, listen with awareness to the sound of *hum*. Continue the technique with total concentration and awareness, listening inwardly to the sound of the mantra and following the movement of *prana* up and down the psychic passage within the spine.

The following is a more advanced technique.

1. As in the previous technique, sit in a meditational posture with your eyes focused calmly at the spiritual eye. Observe the natural flow of the breath with total awareness for a few minutes.
2. Focus your awareness in the psychic passage within the spine, then begin to raise the *prana* (life-force) with the breath through the

NIYAMA 83

inner spinal passage (*sushumna*). The breath should be felt passing consciously through each of the chakras as it ascends and descends through the *sushumna nadi*.

3   In this technique, breathe in *ujjayi pranayama* (see chapter 5). *Ujjayi* helps to induce a deeper meditative state and calms the nervous system down.

   As you inhale, let your throat be open and expanded so that air flowing in through the nasal passages is directed against the back of the throat behind the tongue. This creates a suction effect, pulling the current gently upward. Exhale naturally, allowing the current of energy to descend through the chakras.

4   When you have established a comfortable rhythm of breathing in the spine, synchronize the *soham* mantra with the breath. Again, looking deeply into the spiritual eye and listening with awareness to the sound of the mantra, begin to ascend the *prana* or current of energy through the chakras, from the base chakra (*muladhara*) to the spiritual eye (*ajna chakra*). Be consciously aware of each chakra as you pass through it (see chapter 1). When you reach the spiritual eye hold the breath for three seconds. This can also be practised when you pause at the base of the spine (*muladhara chakra*).

5   Continue until you enter a deep meditative state. Rest in the silent stillness, feeling calmly surrendered in the peace and joy of God.

The Mantra *Om*

The mystic primordial sound *om* is at the root of all mantras. It is the origin of all other sounds and contains all sounds. The cosmic sound of *om* is called in Sanskrit the *pranava* ('sacred syllable').

In the Vedic scriptures, it is said that Brahman (the absolute Reality, pure Consciousness) revealed Itself originally as sound and the first sound was *om*. Therefore *om* is the closest symbol of God for deepening the concentration of the mind, leading to the realization of the supreme Reality.

In the Bible, we read: 'In the beginning was the Word, and the Word was with God, and the Word was God.' (John 1:1) This means that before creation, nothing existed except God the Father as pure spirit: ever-existing, ever-conscious, ever new bliss. God created the universe and everything in it through his Word (which *is* God), the cosmic sound vibration *om* (the Holy Ghost or Holy Spirit). God the Father, or Christ intelligence, guides the cosmic vibration to create all finite matter.

The cosmic vibration of *om* is used by Hindus as *aum*, Muslims as *amin*, and Christians as 'amen'.

Paramhansa Yogananda has said that John the Baptist was baptized by the omnipresent sound of *aum* (the Holy Ghost), and that in a previous incarnation he was Jesus' guru, called Elias. (Matthew 11:13–15 and 17:9–13 demonstrate support for the doctrine of reincarnation.)

Jesus became the Christ after being baptized by his guru, John. In the Bible John says, 'I saw the Spirit descending from heaven like a dove, and it abode upon him [Jesus].' (John 1:32) Potentially, Jesus was a Master from birth, but it was actually at the time of his baptism or initiation by John the Baptist that be become a Master, Jesus the *Christ*. The Word (Holy Ghost or *aum*) had descended into Jesus (symbolized in the Bible and paintings of the baptism as a pure white dove). His human consciousness had expanded with the sound cosmic vibration of *aum*. Jesus embraced the vastness of infinite vibration. His consciousness became identified with the Christ-consciousness, which is the only reflection in all creation of God, the Father beyond creation. 'Christ' means 'the anointed of God' or 'chosen by God'.

The Hindu and Christian Trinity

The mantra *aum–tat–sat* has its equivalent in the Trinity of Christianity.

- *aum (om)* – the Holy Ghost
- *tat* (*kuthastha chaitanya*) – Christ-consciousness (God the Son)
- *sat* – the Father aspect of God, the spirit beyond all vibration

Brahma, Vishnu and Shiva (the Hindu Trinity) do not represent the same aspects as the Christian Trinity, a common mistake made by Western followers of yoga. The triple divinity, Brahma (the Creator), Vishnu (the Preserver) and Shiva (the Destroyer) personify the three aspects of the mantra *aum*.

- *A* represents the creative vibration (Brahma), the manifestation.

Niyama

- *U* represents the preserving vibration (Vishnu), the maintenance.
- *M* represents the destructive vibration (Shiva), the dissolution.

Sounding the *Mantra Aum (Om)*

The mantra *aum* may be sounded aloud, whispered or repeated mentally. The correct pronunciation of the three-syllabled *aum* is *om*, as in the English word, 'home'. The three syllables should be pronounced equally.

In sounding the word, the *a* and the *u* become blended into *o*. The letter *a* starts at the back of the mouth, with the tongue lying relaxed on the lower palate, the sound resonating deeply from the lower abdomen. The letter *u* is formed in the middle of the mouth, and the letter *m* is formed by closing the lips. As the full range of the mouth is used, it is said that *om* contains all sounds.

In the Sanskrit symbol ॐ the crescent (or *nada*) represents the continuing sound prolonged by the person chanting. The dot (or *bindu*) indicates the termination of sound – not a distinct stop but a fading away. The number 3 (important in numerology) is in evidence with the three letters representing the physical, mental and spiritual bodies. Respectively the three letters of *aum* also represent waking consciousness, dream consciousness, and dreamless sleep.

Patanjali in his *Yoga Sutras* suggests *om* as something which reminds us of God. 'The signified meaning of God is *om*.' (1:27) Again, we refer to the Gospel according to St John (1:1):

'In the beginning was the Word, and the Word was with God, and the Word was God.'

God and the Word (*om*) are one and the same. The Word (*om*) is with God now and it will always be with God. It is unchangeable, imperishable and eternal even when the universe and all that is manifested undergo change or dissolution.

In the next sutra, Patanjali instructs us how to use *om*. 'Practise the repetition (*japa*) of *om* and meditate on its meaning with faith and devotion.' (1:28)

To remind you again, *svadhyaya* means self-study. One aspect of self-study is the recitation of mantra. In the above extracts, Patanjali is saying that the mantra *om* be recited only to oneself, which is called *japa*.

Om draws our attention from mental, emotional and physical distractions to superconscious levels of perception. With intensity of concentration on *om* without distraction, all obstacles fall away. The mind then becomes one-pointed, calm and peaceful. In that complete mental tranquillity, there is an experience of great joy.

> One who closes the [nine] doors of the senses and fixes the mind in the heart centre, meditating with life-force in the higher brain centres, who engages in the steady practice of yoga, reciting om, the divine Name that represents the changeless Brahman [God] and remembering Me at the time of death attains the supreme goal.
>
> Bhagavad Gita, 8:12, 13

The following is the technique for chanting *om*.

1. Sit in a comfortable meditative posture. Relax the mind and body and keep the body still. Close the eyes and focus your concentration at the point between the eyebrows, at the spiritual eye.
2. Begin by chanting *om* aloud and feel the vibrations resonating through your whole being. Inhale deeply and let the sound of *om* flow out with the natural exhalation. Continue chanting *om* audibly like this for about ten minutes or more.
3. Now chant *om* in a whisper for about ten minutes.
4. Then, concentrating deeply at the spiritual eye, mentally chant *om*, feeling the vibrations pulsing there. Attentively listen with the inner ear to the sound as you chant (ten minutes).
5. Now be still, enter meditation with your concentration deeply fixed at the spiritual eye, feel your awareness expand into *om*. Contemplate the innate power of the sound of *om* and its spiritual significance.
6. Continue meditating, surrendering into the vibrations of *om*. Feel your awareness expanding still further into the field of pure consciousness, become one with *om*.

Mala Beads

Mala (or rosary) beads are used in counting the number of repetitions of a mantra, Names of God, breaths or *kriyas*.

A *mala* consists of a string of 108 beads. This is a spiritual number: $1 + 0 + 8 = 9$. The number 9 cannot be destroyed, no matter how

NIYAMA 87

many times you multiply it or add it to its own multiple, it is the sacred number of eternity.

The 1 of 108 symbolizes God the Creator. The 0 added to the 1 gives it power and represents God's creation as complete. The number 8 is the symbol for eternity.

Each *mala* of 108 beads has an extra bead offset from the main circle. This bead is called a *sumeru* or Mount Meru, which acts as a reference point, so that the practitioner knows when he or she has completed a rotation of 108 beads.

Mala beads are usually made of sandalwood, rudraksha seeds, tulsi or crystal. Each material has its own particular vibrations. Sandalwood helps to calm the mind and connects the base with the crown chakra. Rudraksha is the fruit of a tree grown in India, Nepal and Java. This is the only fruit in which the stone and the pulp cannot be separated. When the fruit is ripe, the outer pulp becomes dry, wrinkled and very hard. At this stage the seeds can be used for *malas*. Rudraksha has a beneficial influence on the blood circulation, strengthens the heart and is recommended for those who have high blood pressure. Tulsi is a

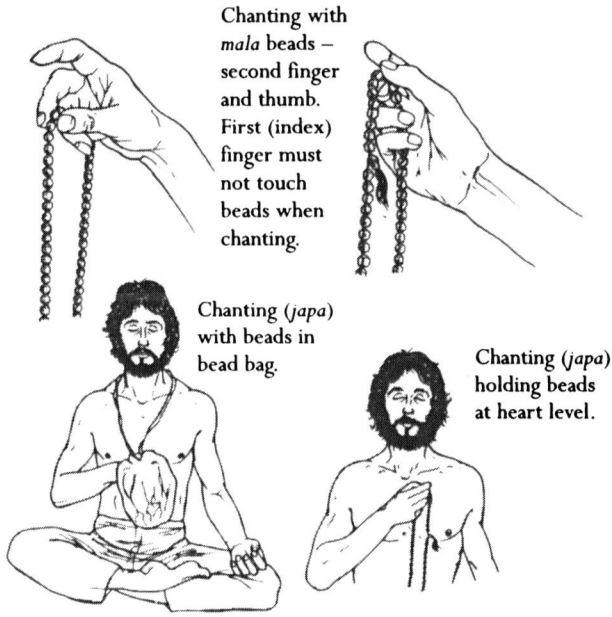

Figure 11 *Chanting with mala beads*

plant related to the herb basil. In India tulsi plants are worshipped by followers of Vishnu and Krishna. The branches of this plant are used for making *malas* and the leaves have medicinal value. Crystal *malas* are used for their psychic properties. Crystal beads can be mixed with rudraksha to add more power. Likewise sandalwood and crystal beads make a good combination for a *mala*.

To use a *mala*, hold the beads in the right hand, between the tip of the thumb and the tip of the middle finger. Do not use the index finger to rotate the beads as it is considered inauspicious in mantra-chanting. Use the middle finger. Start by chanting the mantra on the first bead next to the *sumeru* bead, then rotate the next bead and so on, until you have chanted the mantra on all 108 beads. When you come back to the *sumeru* bead turn the beads and start rotating them in the other direction. You should never chant on the *sumeru* bead or cross over it. Always rotate the *mala* towards the palm.

After your practice you either wear your *mala* around your neck or place it on your altar. Respect it with sacredness; do not let other people touch it.

Using a *mala* helps the mind to concentrate and physically releases nervous and restless energy by the movement of the hand.

Affirmation

I resolve now to live life completely in each moment with inner awareness.

I look and listen attentively with interest to life. With clear understanding, I live centred in soul-awareness.

I observe with awareness from moment to moment my own thoughts, feelings, motives and desires. I identify and renounce those habits that prevent me from giving attention to important priorities, and my true purpose and direction in life.

I keep my mind and senses harmonized with the divine spirit within me by chanting and meditating on God's Name – God and His Name are one.

God is the inner light within my being, which illuminates my path, provides the answers that I seek and guides me to success in all that I think, say or do.

ISVARAPRANIDHANA: SURRENDER TO GOD

'By total surrender to God one attains perfection in God-realization [*samadhi*].' (*The Yoga Sutras of Patanjali*, 2:45) Surrender to God is also referred to by Patanjali in the first part of his sutras (*samadhi-pada*): '*Samadhi* is also obtained by those who surrender to God.' (1:23)
Ishvara means 'the supreme Lord' or 'God'. *Pranidhanat* means 'total surrender'.

As you read the above sutras, the following questions will probably arise in your mind.
1 What stops us from knowing, realizing and experiencing God?
2 Who or what is God?
3 Who surrenders and what is surrendered?

IGNORANCE, THE SELF-LIMITING BARRIER

What stops us from knowing, realizing and experiencing God? The answer is ignorance, which arises in the mind as egotism, the idea of 'I'. Patanjali describes ignorance and egotism in two sutras.

> *Ignorance gives to ego-sense, by identifying with the impermanent as eternal, the impure as pure, the painful as pleasurable, and ego-sense to be the true self.*
>
> Yoga Sutras, 2:5

> *Egotism is the false identification of the seer [soul] with the instrument of seeing [body-mind].*
>
> 2:6

Ignorance begins in the mind, when the sense of 'I' or ego-sense arises. Due to misidentification the ego has forgotten its identity with the supreme Self or God, and has created its own prison.

All the suffering, sorrow and unhappiness we experience in life is not God's fault or doing, but our own. Through ignorance we lose our self-awareness, we forget God. The desire or need for something other than God causes separation from Him. We become divided and separated from our source of ever-new joy, inner peace and divine love, which creates sorrow and unhappiness in us. Until we awaken to our true identity and are united with our Source (God), we will continue to mistakenly identify with the mind, body and senses, causing more unhappiness, restlessness and discontent.

The spirit of God lives within us as pure consciousness, it is our true self, our inner Reality, but until we consciously know, experience and become aware of our Reality we will not succeed in attaining our union with God.

Mind, Ego and Intellect

The human physical brain is not the mind, it is an instrument used by the mind.

You, the individual soul, are *not* the mind, body or senses. You, the soul or Self are pure consciousness, eternally existing. The Self is beyond the characteristics of the mind, body and senses. It is the Self or soul—consciousness that activates and gives life to the mind, body and senses.

The mind is a very subtle form of matter, which appears to be intelligent, but is actually unintelligent. The only source of intelligence in the body is the soul, that is self-illumined. The mind and senses do not shine by their own light, by themselves they are lifeless. The mind and senses receive their life and activity from the soul-consciousness. The soul is always the subject and never the object.

Thought, which arises in the mind, has no intelligence of its own, because its movement is limited by its identity and its own programming. Thought is conditioned by the past and is always a movement away from *what is* in the present moment. The mind is constantly changing, its thoughts weaving backwards and forwards between the past and the future. This constant activity and movement of thought distracts us from being consciously and attentively aware of the present moment.

Thought creates division and disharmony in the mind. When the mind is silent and attentive to the moment, with awareness, it becomes undivided, calm and alert, to perceive and reflect life clearly.

The ego (*ahamkara*) and intellect (*buddhi*) are mental faculties of the mind (*manas*).

The mind receives sensations and impressions from the senses and sends reactions to them; the mind thinks, wills and doubts.

The discriminative and decision-making faculty of the mind is called the intellect. The intellect can judge, understand, compare and explain the objects on the relative plane of existence, but it is a limited instrument and it is unable to gauge the limitless. The intellect cannot know God, who is infinite, who inspires and activates the mind.

The ego is the faculty of identification, both with the objects of the world and with God. The ego is a bridge between the soul and the world. It co-ordinates the physical and mental functions of the human organism. Without the ego, the mind-body would run wild. The ego is necessary for synchronized functioning and harmony within the mind-body as a whole. What causes all the problems is the over-identification of the individual self with the ego. Someone who is egotistic has an extreme amount of self-interest, to the exclusion and detriment of others. An egotistic person acts from a sense of self-aggrandisement, isolation and insecurity. The ego creates its own individuality; it is always looking for new thoughts to continue its existence, it cannot survive without subject-object relation. The ego seeks security in repetition and habit. Its defence is the continuation of thought. When egotism is dominant, awareness is clouded, the light of the soul is unable to shine through.

The ego says 'This is mine', 'I want this, I don't want that', 'I am this body', 'I am this mind'. Its vocabulary consists of 'I', 'me', 'my' and 'mine'. The ego is submerged in its own ignorance, it cannot see God or truth if it is identifying with the mind, body and objects of the senses.

Our true Self will always be falsely represented by the ego until the mind becomes unconditioned from its ignorance. The mind becomes illuminated by Self when it turns inward to investigate its own source and nature.

WITH SURRENDER COMES TRUE FREEDOM

Who surrenders and what is surrendered? Surrender means the surrender of the 'I' or 'ego', or even more appropriately the realization of the non-existence of the ego and that God alone is.

'I' or ego does not surrender something else, therefore surrender is not 'giving away'. Only when there is direct understanding of this truth that God alone is is there surrender. It is the result of non-attachment, selflessness and total dedication to self-awareness from moment to moment, with total trust and acceptance of the present.

Knowledge which is the true Self is veiled by an assumption of the 'I' or ego as an independent entity, but when the light of knowledge shines, the ego is seen to be non-existent. Darkness is an absence of light. We can keep darkness away from a room by switching on a light, but the moment we lose our self-awareness and forget God, the ego, with all its desires and attachments, keeps us in its prison of ignorance.

When the ego is surrendered, the mind becomes still, and in the silent mind God reveals Himself. It is the ego that creates division and restlessness in the mind. There is a very simple but beautiful example to illustrate this fact. When the sun is shining, it is one and unbroken. Let us assume you have a bowl of water and you are looking at the reflection of the sun in it. It is beautifully still, round and radiant. Suddenly the wind blows and the surface of the water is agitated. You then see that the sun has been broken. Even in what is one and indivisible, the agitated mind seems to create a division. As long as the subject-object division exists, the agitation of the mind will continue. When you begin to be aware of the subject and the object together, then the restlessness comes to an end, and with it all our temptations, personal desires, attachments and selfish motives.

Yogis have often given two examples to help us understand the concept of surrender. The first is of a hand between a light and a wall. When you shine your torch on the shadow on the wall, the shadow surrenders itself to the light; it becomes absorbed.

The second example is of a doll made of salt which had the power to think. One day it was standing on the beach and began to think, how big is this ocean and how deep is it? At that moment, there was a boat going to the sea, so the doll jumped on it. The doll looked and looked, and wondered how deep the ocean was at that point. Suddenly, it decided to dive into the ocean to see. As it dived in, it instantly knew and experienced the length, breadth and depth of the ocean; instantly, because when it dissolved it became the ocean. This dissolution is possible because the salt-doll was also made of the ocean salt.

Similarly, there is nothing called 'I' or 'me' which is other than the universe. The body is made of the material elements of the universe – earth, water, fire, air, ether. Air is moving throughout the body to keep it alive. There is also intelligence of course, which is also of the universe. In the *Bhagavad Gita* (7:4, 5), Lord Krishna informs us: 'Earth, water, fire, air, ether, mind, intelligence and false ego – altogether these eight comprise My separated material energies.' The subtle body is comprised of the mind, intelligence and false ego, which is also of a lower, inferior nature to the superior nature of the self. What is it that I consider 'me'? An examination of the self in this manner is also called surrender.

Self-realization means realizing your true self as the great ocean of spirit, by breaking the delusion that you are this little ego, this little human body and personality.

Paramhansa Yogananda, from *The Essence of Self-Realization* by Sri Kriyananda

To know complete surrender, look at and study the lives of past saints and Masters like Jesus Christ, St Francis of Assisi, Sri Anandamayi Ma, Paramhansa Yogananda and others. You will see that their lives were an offering at the feet of God; for them there was only God.

Mother Teresa of Calcutta is an outstanding example of one who is totally surrendered in love and devotion to God and in serving others in God. Love and service go together, the fulfilment of love is service. When we surrender to this divine love within us, we become embodiments of that love.

WHO OR WHAT IS GOD?

To truly understand what God is, we need to transcend the mind. Mind is matter, subject to change. It is limited and conditioned by thought. The limited material mind cannot understand God, who is unlimited, infinite and more subtle than mind. We cannot know and experience God with the mind, merely by intellectualizing or reading books about it. We have to transcend the mind/ego/intellect and let go of all concepts of what God is.

In the beginning of our search for God, thinking and reading about God may help us to open ourselves consciously to inner awareness. But first we must honestly and willingly admit that all our knowledge about God has come through the opinions, concepts and thoughts of the limited, finite human mind.

The mind cannot know that which is beyond the mind. We have to transcend the mind by quietening it, by stilling our thoughts. In that stillness, where the constant chattering of the mind ceases, we remain in the conscious awareness of the Self and listen attentively. It is in this inner stillness that God reveals Himself as inner joy, inner peace, inner love and wisdom. Knowing God comes from inner soul-realization. We, the individual soul, are made in the image and likeness of God, so, when we are consciously aware of His presence within us and commune with God, we experience those manifestations and qualities which are God divine love, divine joy, wisdom, inner light and inner peace. In deep meditation in inner communion with God one is able to experience God as the cosmic sound vibration (the Holy Ghost) of *om*.

The soul is aware of its divinity; it intuitively feels itself to be eternal as God is, and that in oneness with God it manifests those very same qualities that God manifests.

We are all seeking pure love, inner peace and ever-new joy, but due to forgetfulness and ignorance we are not consciously aware of our true nature as the ever-existing, ever-conscious, blissful soul within. Due to our unawareness and ignorance we unsuccessfully strive to find peace, love and joy outwardly through the limited mind, body and senses.

Many of us never seem to learn that our freedom, peace, love and joy are not dependent on outer conditions and circumstances. We have become so conditioned by our minds and by our thoughts that we are unaware God is closer to us than our own breath. God is *not* separate and apart from us. He is not sitting disinterestedly in some far corner of the universe, withholding His love. He is *not* a cruel and vengeful God giving out punishments and diseases to those that have sinned and blessings only to those who are good. God neither wills nor sends disease as punishment. From beginning to end God is clearly revealed in the Bible, particularly the New Testament, as a loving and healing God. His whole purpose, we are told, is to bring all things to wholeness. The divine plan is one of renewal, restoration and perfection. God did not create us to be diseased. We were made to be perfect in mind, body and spirit, and to be full of love, joy, peace, wisdom and health. There is no warrant in the scriptures for believing that disease is part of God's plan, any more than sin is. God did not create it, nor does He purposely inflict it upon us. God made all things good, and God in all His goodness is within each and every one of us. God is truth, and all that is good is from Him, of Him, and in Him.

Truth is always positive and creative, it is the light that is hidden by the ignorance of the ego and selfishness in our hearts. It is our negative thoughts such as fear, anxiety, worry, anger, hatred, resentment and jealousy that deny the truth that God loves us and that His love is part of the life in us, working in us for our good. When we hold on to these negative thoughts, we deny the actuality of God's qualities in us, of love, peace, calmness, joy and contentment.

Truth is infinite. No religion, cult, sect, or organization has an exclusive authority to represent truth. No one can have the last word about it because truth cannot be organized, it is not static, it is always new in every moment; it is unlimited. The ignorant, selfish and power-hungry mind tries to crystallize truth by organizing it with narrow creeds and dogma, but truth cannot and will not be confined within the walls of error.

God is love and God is forever expressing His love to all life in His creation, in this universe. Everything that exists does so because God's life, God Himself, is in it. God is the author and giver of life and without the life that God is, creation would dissolve and there would be nothing. 'In Him we live and move and have our being.' (Acts 17:28) God also lives and has being in us.

God's love, which caused all creation, cannot rest content with anything less than perfection, and so is constantly working towards it. God is greater than His creation, but He is also in it. God is transcendent, beyond His world, but He is also immanent, remaining in the midst of it. Our purpose is to co-operate with God's Will and be willing instruments through which truth can reveal itself, to be a perfect channel through which God's Will may be done, by attuning ourselves to God and realizing our oneness with Him. Our lives are also intended for the selfless service of all. Through selfless service we expand the heart and break all barriers that stand in the way of the unity and oneness of all existence. Selfless service with love opens the heart and purifies the mind. Both meditation and service are important to practise if we are to progress quickly along the spiritual path.

Our purpose is to co-operate with God's Will, but we are given free choice to act as we will. We can either make ourselves one with God, or separate ourselves from Him. Our suffering, sorrow, unhappiness and disease are brought upon us by our own ignorance and forgetfulness of God. We cause our own suffering through our unawareness of God, by thinking that our purpose here on earth is to gratify our own selfish desires, without thinking of what God's desire is, what God wants us to do, what God's Will is for us.

Paramhansa Yogananda said:

Human suffering is not a sign of God's anger with mankind. It is a sign, rather, of man's ignorance of the divine law. The law is forever infallible in its workings.

From *The Essence of Self-Realization* by Sri Kriyananda

God is not changeable. Being the great authority behind and in all things, He works, as indeed any other lesser authority does, by the rule of law. For example, a government brings the rule of beneficent law to its people. If the law is broken then the people suffer. Similarly, if we break God's immutable laws, we cease to enjoy the fulness of His goodness, even while it is within our grasp.

Every action and every thought reaps its own corresponding rewards. The natural law of cause and effect is immutable and operates everywhere in the physical world and on the mental plane. Things do not happen in this world, or even in this universe, by accident or by chance. There is a reason and a positive, definite cause behind everything that happens, whether it be diseases of the body, earthquakes, floods, volcanic eruptions, the outbreak of war, a plane or car crash, rising to fame and becoming rich, or losing all to become homeless on the streets.

This natural law of causation is known as the doctrine or law of *karma*. *Karma* is a Sanskrit word meaning any kind of mental or physical action, and the result of an action. These actions are imprinted in the mind and are called *samskaras* (impressions). Our past *samskaras* motivate our present actions; what we sow is what we reap.

Paramhansa Yogananda once enlightened a disciple on *karma*.

'It seems unfair,' a disciple lamented, 'that we should be punished for mistakes that we made unintentionally, without realizing they were wrong.'

'Ignorance,' replied the Master, 'doesn't alter the law. If a person drives his car absent-mindedly into a tree, his resulting injuries won't be fewer because he was absent-minded.

'You must learn to adapt your actions to the law. As Sri Yukteswarji [Yogananda's guru] remarked once to me, "The cosmos would be fairly chaotic if its laws could not operate without the sanction of human belief."'

From *The Essence of Self-Realization* by Sri Kriyananda

We create our own happiness or unhappiness by our own thoughts and actions. Both man and woman are that which they will themselves to be. Our whole character is determined by the thoughts for which we allow a place in our mind. Strong people are what they are because of repeated thoughts of strength. Every act and every condition has its origin in the mind. Thoughts, whether positive or negative, are seeds that, when dropped or planted in the subconscious mind, germinate, grow and bring forth their fruit in due season.

No one, including God, is responsible for our thoughts and actions but ourselves. It is our very own mind that is the cause of our suffering and unhappiness, it creates all our feelings and experiences of pain and pleasure.

God is love. Love never hurts or destroys, for like all good qualities, love is creative. God gives His love equally to all, He is all-benevolent and all-loving. God is not a fearful God, we have no need to fear Him, for fear only keeps us away from Him. The correct way to approach God is just as a child would approach its mother, with complete trust and love. God is like the mother, loving, kind, forgiving and protective against all harm.

In the Bible, St Paul beautifully describes to us what love is:

> *Love is patient, love is kind. It does not envy, it does not boast, it is not proud. It is not rude, it is not self-seeking, it is not easily angered, it keeps no record of wrongs. Love does not delight in evil but rejoices with the truth. It always protects, always trusts, always hopes, always preserves. Love never fails.*
>
> 1 Corinthians 13:4–8

It is through love that we can approach God and draw inspiration from Him by offering our hearts unconditionally to Him.

The best way by which we can show our love for God is by constant remembrance of Him, not only in meditation but in all our daily activities. If we forget God, then our love is lost, we feel a separation from that inner joy, inner calmness and peace without knowing why. When we forget God and feel separated, our minds become restless and run from one thing to another in pursuit of objects of the senses outside, instead of looking within in the stillness of the heart to that supreme Reality, whose nature is ever-new joy, love and peace.

We need to practise the presence of God. This involves establishing a continuing awareness of God with love, trust, faith and devotion, in every aspect of our lives. It is turning our thoughts from outer circumstances to the presence of God within.

If we feel distant from God, it is because we have created the distance. When we bring our awareness and attention back to God, the source of all joy, love, peace, knowledge and wisdom, feelings of separation disappear.

Before we can practise the presence of God, we must first come to know God. How we relate to God is determined by our understanding of Him.

The sacred scriptures and saints and sages tell us what God is.

> *God is not far from each one of us. For in Him we live and move and have our being.*
>
> Acts 17:27-8

> *God is love and anyone who lives in love lives in God, and God lives in him.*
>
> 1 John 4:16

> *God is Spirit.*
>
> 1 John 4:24

> *God is Light.*
>
> 1 John 1:5

> *God is Eternal.*
>
> Genesis 21:33

> *In the beginning was the Word, and the Word was with God and the Word was God.*
>
> John 1:1

Paramhansa Yogananda has said that the Word (Holy Ghost) is the cosmic intelligent sound vibration *om*.

The yogic scriptures tell us that God is *satchitananda* (ever-existing, ever-conscious, ever-new bliss), meaning that God's joy is ever-new.

In the *Brahma-Sutras*, an ancient Vedic scripture, God is explained as Him from whom everything emanates. The Supreme Being is fully cognisant of everything, directly and indirectly; unless He is fully cognisant of everything, He cannot be God.

Both the *Bhagavad Gita* and the Bible tell us that God is ever-living and eternal.

> *Never was there a time when I did not exist, nor you, nor all these things, nor in the future shall any of us cease to be.*
>
> Bhagavad Gita 2:12

NIYAMA 99

> *'I am the Alpha and the Omega,' says the Lord God, 'who is, and who was, and who is to come, the Almighty.'*
>
> Revelations, 1:8

Eternity into the past seems impossible for us to comprehend fully, and yet, beyond the farthest reaches of our imagination, God has always been.

Even if we think that someone else created God, this still implies the existence of an ultimate cause.

No one made God because God, and God only, as the First Cause, is the cause of everything that is made. Whereas we come into existence only when something causes us to exist, *God simply is*. God *is* even before the beginning.

Admitting an ultimate cause, we must ask the basic question of creation: was that original cause conscious or inert?

We wonder at the creation and workings of nature. What is the power that produces a huge tree with twigs, leaves, flowers and fruit from a tiny seed? What is the power that supplies water for trees, flowers and the food that grows on this earth? At whose command does the sun rise to give warmth, light and energy? The sun and rain bring life to the plant and tree from without, but inside it are the tiny cells, perfectly adapted to their work, absorbing and distributing the sustenance. The life of God is in them all, sun, rain and cells. It is invisible, intangible and it cannot be magnified, dissected or analysed, but there it is, and neither sun nor rain nor cells would be of any use without it.

Who divided the seasons and changes the colour of the leaves on the trees in autumn? Look at the vastness of space above you: there is a perfect orchestrated order to it. The planets revolve on a precise degree of axis and at an exact speed; if they were to do otherwise the universe would be in chaos, there would be no order. Is this then a display of intelligent creation or a product of a fortuitous combination of particles of matter?

God is the all-prevading spirit and life of the universe, He is the essential power and reality in all things. God is the first causeless cause, whose conscious Will rules every action in the universe.

> *I am the Source of all spiritual and material worlds. Everything emanates from Me.*
>
> Bhagavad Gita 10:8

> *Of all creations I am the beginning, the end and also the middle.*
>
> Bhagavad Gita 10:32

The difficulty we have in accepting something or someone without a cause is due to our conditioned life, for nothing within our experience has ever been causeless.

There are some people who think of God as being some kind of void or empty vacuum, but even in outer space there is an ethereal ocean of waves, rays, particles, light and sound vibrations. All over the universe there are innumerable planets and stars. Our own planet contains mountains, rivers, birds, animals, trees, plants and people – people with feelings, ideas and creativity. Since God by definition is the source of all that exists, our conception must be adequate to explain how He has caused all these manifestations. How could so many human beings and other forms at different levels of consciousness come from a void, from nothing?

God is the Supreme Intelligence that gave birth to all life. First came God's conscious vibratory consciousness, out of which unfolded, through cosmic sound vibration and cosmic light, the causal, astral and material worlds.

The material objects were formed by the condensing of the subtlest of elements down through to the grossest, in the following order: ether, air, fire, water, earth.

Are we God? In essence we are, for we are an eternal part of Him. God is not separate from us, He is omnipresent, He is the divine indweller within us all. Although in quality we are the same as God, we cannot be greater than God. The emanations cannot have or be more than the whole.

> *The soul (jivatma) in the body is a part of My eternal Self; it attracts to itself the mind and the five senses, which rest in matter (prakriti).*
>
> Bhagavad Gita 15:7

> *You are the Father, also the greatest teacher of this animate and inanimate creation and supremely adorable. You are the possessor of incomparable glory, in all the three worlds there is no one equal to You; how can anyone be superior?*
>
> Bhagavad Gita 11:43

Although religion generally teaches that we are all eternal, most of the world scriptures make the distinction between the infinite greatness of God and the infinitesimal nature of God's eternal parts (the individual souls). If you, I and everyone else are God, why can we not create an entire cosmic universe? If I am God why do I have to suffer the miseries of disease, old age and death in this material body? If I am God, but have forgotten, how did I forget? Forgetfulness implies that the force of ignorance (*avidya*) or illusion (*maya*) is more powerful than me. That means that I am not God, for God is not subject to ignorance or illusion, He is without pain, pleasure, sorrow and fear. 'God is Light; in Him there is no darkness at all.' (1 John 1:5)

It is only the 'I' or false ego that is subject to ignorance and illusion. Although God is immanent in the world, God is also transcendental, He rises above it. God can never be polluted or coloured by ignorance.

As the material elements enter the bodies of all living beings and yet remain outside them all, I exist within all material creations and yet am not within them.

Srimad Bhagavatam 2:9:35

Does God have form or is God formless?

God is impersonal in His formless aspect, but in His personal or manifest aspect he is love. The great Masters, saints and avatars are the incarnations or forms of God as love. Jesus Christ, Lord Krishna, Buddha, St Francis of Assisi and Paramhansa Yogananda are some of the shining examples of God's love in form. These great lights that come into the world to illumine the darkness and show us God's love were also the impersonal infinite consciousness behind the form.

God can be realized as formless (*nirguna*) or with form (*saguna*), they are inseparably linked. God is beyond form and yet He takes on all forms. God is omnipotent, He can be in the atom and simultaneously in the vast universe.

Although the sun stays in one part of the universe, still it is simultaneously present everywhere in its expansion of sunshine. Just as the energy and the energetic cannot be separated, so it is the same with God and His creation.

Since God is omnipresent, He has also assumed the form of the universe. The whole universe is an expression of God's love. God reveals to us His love and wisdom through the beauty He has created in the numerous and varied forms around us in the world and universe.

When we feel close to nature we can feel, see and experience God's love and beauty in the flowers, plants and trees – these are expressions of the delicacy, sensitiveness and gentleness of His life-force.

Is God one or many? God is one without a second, there is no other God besides Him. All of us as individual souls are numerous reflected souls of the one universal spirit (God).

In this universe there is only one sun that gives warmth, light and energy to this planet Earth, there is no other. Similarly there is only one God who shines his divine light, divine love, cosmic energy, and continually showers us with His divine grace.

It is God that dreamed us into existence, His one and only purpose is to see that all His children evolve spiritually.

God belongs to no religion, church or organization and yet He belongs to all, because God is everywhere and He is everything. God is formless and at the same time He is the form of all forms.

God is worshipped in different religions by different names according to the characteristic or quality to which a person wishes to express their devotion and aspiration. In India for example, God is worshipped through many gods and goddesses, which are simply seen and experienced as different manifestations of the one absolute truth. Each deity embodies a particular aspect or quality of the Supreme. For example, Brahma, Vishnu and Shiva are the three aspects of God. Brahma is the creative aspect, Vishnu is the preserving aspect, and Shiva is the destructive or dissolving aspect.

There is a wonderful little story of a holy man who lived in India during the 16th century, who asked for forgiveness for the three errors he had committed during the life of his devotional practices.

- He gave God a name and a conceptual form – God who cannot be limited to names, concepts or form – but the holy man needed to do so in order to relate his limited mind through a relatable means.
- He worshipped God in a temple – God who is everywhere and cannot be confined to any one place – but he needed to go to a sacred place to find peace and quiet.
- He glorified God who, unlike the human ego, seeks no glorification, but he did so to be humble and transcend his ego by attributing to God all that there was to be grateful about.

The Lord our God is one Lord.

Deuteronomy 6:4

There is one God; and there is no other than He.

Mark 12:32

I am the source of all creation. Everything in the world moves because of Me; with this realization the wise, full of devotion, worship Me.

Bhagavad Gita 10:8

Arjuna, even those devotees who, endowed with faith, worship other gods, they too worship Me alone, without proper knowledge. For I am the only enjoyer and Lord of all sacrifices. Those who are deluded and fail to realize My true nature are subjected to birth and death.

Those who worship the gods (devas) go to the gods; those who worship their ancestors, and those who worship ghosts find their place with them, but those who worship Me attain Me.

Bhagavad Gita 9:23-5

God is one, there can be no separateness from Him. God is both manifest and unmanifest, He manifests in all He has created, from the mineral, plant and animal kingdoms to human beings. The only separateness is from our own ignorance. Our delusion of separateness causes us to see diversity in the world.

If you have the wisdom of God-consciousness, then you will see God and God alone everywhere.

Ramana Maharshi

The yogi who is united in identity with the all-pervading infinite consciousness, sees the Self abiding in all beings and all beings in the Self; he sees the same everywhere.

Bhagavad Gita 6:29

He who, established in unity, worships Me as residing in all beings (as their very Self) whatever his mode of existence, realizes Me as pervading all beings.

Bhagavad Gita 6:31

'But to each one of us grace has been given.' (Ephesians 4:7) God's grace is like the sunshine. When clouds come between us and the sun, we cannot feel its warmth or receive its light, but when the clouds are removed we receive its warmth, light and energy. Similarly, God is continually showering us with His grace. We have only to remove the obstructions which make us feel separate from God's energy to experience His loving grace.

God's grace is always available to us. God is within us, and it is God's grace that is our sufficiency in all things. 'My grace is sufficient for you for my power is made perfect in weakness.' (Corinthians 12:9)

It is God's grace that makes us long for Him, and by longing for God we develop a constant remembrance of Him. Through constant remembrance of God, one develops dispassion towards the world and comes closer to God. Dispassion is not rejecting or renouncing life, but living life with complete awareness in God. It is bringing the consciousness of God into all our everyday actions, into everything we do.

We cannot attain God without His grace; remembrance of God comes through His grace.

To be in attunement with God we need to make a deep, conscious meditative effort toward living in the inner awareness of God-consciousness, offering ourselves up with love to the divine and bringing that awareness more into our lives.

Sincerity, self-surrender, love, devotion, conscious awareness, a strong desire to know God and a constant, consistent effort to progress spiritually will bring us more in attunement with God's grace. When we become surrendered in selfless love and selfless service we will feel the reality of divine grace working in our lives at all times. Surrender and grace are interrelated: surrender begins the process of purifying the heart and grace completes it. The more we surrender unconditionally, the more grace we receive.

God's grace comes to us in inner strength, inner peace, understanding and wisdom to overcome obstacles and difficulties. With God's grace the universe meets all our natural needs.

When the disciple is ready the guru appears. When we are sincere in wanting to know God by making a sincere and strong effort to find Him, His divine grace directs us to a saint, guru or Master – a pure, illumined soul who can awaken us from within to realize our divinity. Such saints act as a channel for God in the awakening of mankind to the awareness and consciousness of God.

Attain this truth by approaching a self-realized Master. Surrender to him and with respect and devotion enquire with a sincere heart, and render service to him. The wise seer of truth will unfold that knowledge to you. Then you will no more be subjected to delusion; you will see all beings in the Self and Me.

Bhagavad Gita 4:34-5

The intense desire for God-realization is itself the way to it.

Sri Anandamayi Ma

The Need for Faith in God

The word 'faith' originally comes from a Hebrew root *mn*, from which we derive the word 'amen' ('it is so'). It referred originally to a mother nursing her child. Her arms were secure, safe, trustworthy, they were faithful.

Everybody has some faith, no matter how little, because without it we would not be able to accomplish anything. We must have faith in ourselves and in others to complete any act, whether it be asking our parents when we were born, sitting in the dentist's chair, waiting for the sun to rise or the full moon to appear, or for the decorator to make a good job of decorating the living room.

We need faith in ourselves to achieve our aims and goals. Similarly we need faith in God if we are to progress and unfold spiritually. Faith in yourself and faith in God are actually the same, because your self is God. We forget until that inner faith is called upon suddenly against an enemy without or even an unseen enemy in the form of a disease like cancer. Then your faith in God within is remembered, you draw upon its strength to fight the enemy. Faith in God brings peace of mind, inner strength, courage and wisdom to face the everyday storms and trials in life. Faith in God gives deep feelings of assurance, inner security and freedom. When we doubt ourselves then we doubt the God within us, which makes us unsteady and subject to fear and anxiety.

Our true security is in God; when we cultivate our faith in God we shall have a secure foundation on which hope can be built. No matter what trials come to us we will be able to face them all with inner faith and the inner strength of knowing that God's all-embracing love, peace, strength and healing power are with us always.

> *Faith means expanding your intuitive awareness of God's presence within and not relying on reason as your chief means of understanding.*
>
> Paramhansa Yogananda, from *The Essence of Self-Realization* by Sri Kriyananda

Have faith in God.

Jesus Christ in Mark 11:22

Devotion: The Way of Love

> *In the quest for God, the unfolding of the heart's natural love, in the form of deep devotion, is the prime requisite for success. Without devotion, not a single step can be taken towards Him.*
>
> *Devotion is no sentiment: it is the deep longing to commune with, and know, the only Reality there is.*

Sri Kriyananda

Devotion is the surrendered, undivided, loving contemplation of God. The easiest way to transcend or reduce the ego and surrender to the divine Will, is through devotion to God.

The path of knowledge (*jnana*) without love and devotion can be dry and barren. The devotional path (*bhakti*) without knowledge can result in emotional fervour and sentimentality. Both these paths can lead to enlightenment, but the more soul-satisfying path is that which combines self-enquiry and discrimination with loving devotion to God.

One who is truly devoted to God considers every action as service of God and feels the presence of the divine everywhere. The devotee of God loves all beings as manifestations of God himself.

The devotee develops intense longing for and continuous remembrance of God and, through that devoted intensity, merges in God and realizes that 'The Father and I are one.'

When we open ourselves to God and make a sincere effort to know Him, His grace flows to us, and our devotion deepens. Opening to God is not a passive thing, like opening a window and then hoping that the sun is shining. We have to put out a magnetic call to God and attune ourselves to His flow of grace. If we want God, then we have to invite Him into our lives.

God has everything. There really is not anything that he needs from us, except our love. This is the one thing He does not have unless we choose to give it.

When you love someone very deeply, then there is no question of scheduling time for them. The urge to be with your loved one is so great that 'everything else can wait but I must see my beloved'. Similarly, we have to develop a great depth of love for God.

Devotional love can be awakened in us through the association with saints and self-realized gurus, those who have already developed this great depth of love. These saints or Masters may come to you in different ways: in person or through superconscious dreams. You may also associate with the saints by reading about them or feeling their presence in prayer and meditation.

Devotion can also be awakened in us through chanting or singing God's Name (*kirtan*). Paramhansa Yogananda said, 'Chanting is half the battle.' He defined chanting as a singing prayer, or talking to God in devotional song.

Chanting has the power to uplift the mind and heart and turn them toward God. It also has the power to heal the body, mind and soul, but most important is the power chanting has to open our hearts in love and devotion. It is love alone that is the price for admission to God's presence and if we chant His Name with love, sincerity and devotion, He will shower His grace upon us.

Through devotion we develop humility and our loving surrender to God draws Him closer to us.

Fix your mind on Me, be devoted to Me, with ceaseless worship bow reverently before Me. Entering into such complete divine communion you will surely come to Me.

Bhagavad Gita 9:34

The path of love is the highest path. Love of God is supreme; devotion to God is devotion to eternal truth.

Narada Sutras 81

THE PRACTICE OF *ISVARAPRANIDHANA*

1 **Surrender your ego thoughts, ego behaviour, ego attitudes and states of consciousness which are not helpful in unfolding towards self-realization.**

2 Choose a lifestyle which fully supports your highest aspirations, spiritual awareness and total health in mind, body and spirit.

Then live from a higher understanding, to experience your true reality.

3 Make a dedicated inner resolve and affirmation.

Affirm the importance of knowing God, and dedicate yourself to be loyal to your chosen spiritual path.

With unwavering attention and willing participation, make a constant effort to be surrendered in God. Be patient in the face of obstacles and challenges. Have faith and trust in God and your guru to guide you from within.

4 Live with purpose, awareness and understanding.

Open yourself to life by giving and sharing – keep the energy flowing!

5 Cultivate an increased awareness of the presence and reality of God.

6 Meditate regularly and deeply.

Do so with a surrendered heart, love and devotion, to experience a conscious loving relationship with God.

7 Develop trust, faith and devotion in God.

If you do so, surrender will follow. Pray regularly with a surrendered heart in devotion, so that you become aware of God's omnipresence and attract His grace.

8 Raise your consciousness to a higher awareness and understanding during your daily activities.

In all that you do, perform your duties with the thought of God. When duties are performed as an offering to God, it is as spiritually beneficial as meditation.

9 Self-surrender is the result of constant God-remembrance.

10 Understand that God can be loved with or without form.

Attune your mind and will to the divine Will.

11 Associate with others who are devoted to God.

This means especially saints and self-realized gurus, because they are the messengers of God who deny delusion and can awaken in your consciousness the consciousness of God.

12 Sing and chant to God.

This will awaken your soul qualities of love, ever-new joy and devotion to God.

13 Study the lives of great saints, gurus and enlightened Masters.

Read and study spiritually inspiring books such as:
- the *Bhagavad Gita* (especially chapter 12, which focuses on the supreme importance of devotion and faith in spiritual development)
- *Autobiography of a Yogi* by Paramhansa Yogananda
- the New Testament of the Bible
- *Practising the Presence of God* by Brother Lawrence
- *God Alone* by Sister Gyanamata

AFFIRMATION

I release all attachments and desires.

I surrender my ego to my own inner divinity, the spirit of God within. I attune my will to God's Will. Divine intelligence guides me in higher ways of expression. I have complete faith in the presence, love, power, wisdom and life of God.

Through an ever-increasing awareness of the spirit of God within, I am reborn into a consciousness of ever-new joy, inner peace and all-encompassing love, by which I am renewed, revitalized and refreshed.

The love of God surrounds me, I am secure in God's love, strength and peace. From the presence and power of God within, I live, move and have my being. Surrendered in God-realization I am free from the darkness of limitation and delusion. I awake into the light of true freedom, peace, love and ever-new joy!

4

ASANA

Having thoroughly covered *yama* and *niyama* we now come to Patanjali's third limb, *Asana*, which means 'posture' or 'seat'.

Although it is popular now in the West to practise many different yoga postures (Hatha Yoga), Patanjali deals with the subject in only three sutras (2:46–8), and does not name one. In the first of these sutras he says: 'Posture is an attitude in which the body is kept steady (motionless), while producing a feeling of ease.' (*Yoga Sutras* 2:46)

This sutra was prescribed by Patanjali because he mentions in another sutra: 'Unsteadiness of the body or its limbs is an indication of the unsteadiness of the mind.'

Patanjali's description of *asana* does not refer to any particular yoga postures, but only to the ability to hold the body motionlessly still in preparation for, and sitting for long periods in, deep meditation. If the body is restless, then the mind will also become restless. So, in order to ensure that the mind becomes still and quiet, the body needs to be trained, to make it steady with ease and comfort.

A sign of perfection in *asana* is to be able to sit in one place completely motionless and relaxed for three hours. With both the body and the mind stilled, one is able to go deep into meditation and experience calmness, inner peace and inner joy. He says: 'Posture is mastered by freeing the body and mind from tension and restlessness and meditating on the infinite ... When posture is mastered, one is undisturbed by the pairs of opposites (dualities).' (*Yoga Sutras* 2:47–48)

In these sutras he informs us that when we have mastered posture by being steadily seated with both the mind and body in an alert, effortless, relaxed condition, free from restlessness, the mind is then free to meditate on the Infinite. The mind becomes one-pointed and flows in one direction. It is not distracted by the dualities of thought processes and their associations, such as heat and cold, joy and sorrow, pain and pleasure or success and failure.

What is Hatha Yoga?

The Sanskrit word *hatha* consists of two letters, *ha* meaning 'sun' and *tha* meaning 'moon'. The sun refers to the positive, heating, male energy principle in the body, associated with the flow of breath through the right nostril (*pingala*). The moon refers to the negative, cooling, female energy principle, associated with the flow of breath through the left nostril (*ida*). When you have to do something active, you need to have the predominant flow of breath in the right nostril. When you are more reflective or doing something passive the predominant flow of breath should be in the left nostril. With practice it is possible to change the flow of breath mentally from one nostril to the other. For meditation you need the breath flowing evenly through both nostrils.

The aim of Hatha Yoga is to balance, integrate and harmonize these two energy flows in the body, resulting in mental calm, vitality and inner balance.

Hatha Yoga is a complete discipline and practice for the harmonious development of the entire being. It is concerned primarily with preparing the body and mind for the higher spiritual practices and stages of *dharana–dhyana–samadhi* (concentration–meditation–blissful union with God).

The *Hatha Yoga Pradipika*, a 15th-century treatise on the practice of Hatha Yoga by Svatmarama specifically states that Hatha Yoga is a preparation for Raja Yoga (the royal path or yoga of meditation).

It is also the aim of Hatha Yoga to purify the physical body from all toxins, waste matter and disease; to free the body and mind from tensions, and to make the body strong, firm and supple, so that it will remain seated in one position, steadily and comfortably, relaxed for extended periods of time in meditation. Without securing a comfortable, relaxed, steady posture, one cannot progress in meditation.

The *Gheranda Samhita*, another major text of antiquity on Hatha Yoga by Yogi Gheranda, gives six main practices in preparing for the superconscious state of *samadhi*, and the stages attained by practising them.

- purification by regular practice of the six *shat kriyas: dhauti, neti, vasti, tratak, nauli* and *kapalabhati*
- strength by the practice of *asanas*
- steadiness by the practice of *mudras*
- calmness by the practice of *pratyahara*
- lightness by the practice of *pranayama*
- perception by the practice of *meditation*

There are four main classical treatises on Hatha Yoga:

- the *Shiva Samhita*: late 17th century
- the *Gheranda Samhita*: Yogi Gheranda, 15th century
- the *Goraksha Samhita*: Yogi Gorakshanath, 11th century
- the *Hatha Yoga Pradipika*: Yogi Svatmarama, 15th century

Of these four, the *Gheranda Samhita* and the *Hatha Yoga Pradipika* are the two principal ones.

According to the *Hatha Yoga Pradipika*, Lord Shiva (the lord of the yogis) is the founder of Hatha Yoga. He taught all the 84,000 *asanas* to his consort, Parvati. Throughout the centuries this great science has been passed down in disciplic succession. Lord Shiva initiated Matsyendranath, who in turn taught his disciple, Gorakshanath and so on. The *Hatha Yoga Pradipika* lists 35 great Hatha Yoga masters (great *siddhas*). As time went by the many thousands of *asanas* were greatly reduced and modified, until there were no more than a few hundred, of which only 84 are generally known and are of importance. Out of these, only 32 are thought to be commonly useful today.

The oldest known evidence of Hatha Yoga being practised dates back to about 2500 BC. In archaeological excavations at Mohenjo-Daro, a north Indian civilization, a fired clay seal belonging to the ancient Indus Valley civilization (Chalcolithic Age) was found, which is often pointed to as an indication of how old the science of Hatha Yoga really is. It portrays a three-faced human figure sitting in the meditative *asana, bhadrasana* (auspicious posture) – the ankles are placed under the buttocks on either side of the perineum and the soles of the feet are pressed together. This posture is also called *gorakshasana*.

The true purpose of yoga postures and other yoga practices is to awaken and harmonize the inner source of energy, and direct it toward the higher brain centres, to expand one's awareness and consciousness of God.

Hatha Yoga is a wonderful system for attaining perfect health, but the yogi is not really interested in that; he or she does not practise yoga postures just to be healthy. The yogi values health only to the extent that the body should not disturb or distract the mind in its quest for truth or God. The yogi finds a balance in life; he or she does not want to become a health-conscious fanatic or faddist.

Patanjali specifically states in his sutras that ill health is an obstacle to spiritual progress, because if the body is not in a good state of health it will create psychological disturbance in the mind, which will make one's search for truth extremely difficult.

The mind and its mental attitudes influence and affect the body positively or negatively. Conversely, the body and bodily postures influence the mind. The practice of Hatha Yoga re-establishes physical and mental equilibrium in the individual, creating a harmonious flow of energy in the body and mind as one integrated whole.

Hatha Yoga practice removes tension, toxins and impurities and releases energy blocks, which impede the harmonious flow of energy in the body. It promotes perfect health, rejuvenation and longevity. It is to our advantage to live a healthy, long life, because it enables us to fulfil our worthy purposes and to awaken, learn and grow spiritually. The highest purpose and aim in life is to know, love and serve God – to be Self-realized.

With the mind and body in a harmonious, balanced, healthy condition, one is more useful in helping others and serving humanity. In service we consider the needs of others. Through service we learn to see God in all people and all things. Service expands our vision beyond the narrow limits of the ego, and the joy of service is its own reward.

The system of Hatha Yoga co-ordinates the physical and mental aspects of the individual being through conscious control, discipline and awareness of the body and mind. It also teaches the physical body to function efficiently with the minimum consumption of energy. The physical body wastes a great deal of energy, but Hatha Yoga reduces this wastage to the minimum so that more energy can be directed to the attainment of the higher states of consciousness, in which lies the fundamental aim of the yoga system.

The advanced Hatha Yoga student reveals the benefits of yoga and the inner changes that have subtly taken place over some years of practice by the following characteristics: calm, steady gaze; sparkling, aware eyes; soft, mellow, resonant voice; clear skin; strong, firm, supple body; exuberance of vitality and energy; the radiation of joy; emotional and mental balance; complete lack of restlessness in the position and bearing of the body; awareness and alertness, good concentration; a positive, enthusiastic attitude; cheerfulness; physical and mental relaxation; good digestion; and good elimination.

The physical practice of Hatha Yoga consists of:

- the *shatkarmas* – the six purification techniques
- *asanas* – postures
- *mudras* – 'seals' to awaken and direct the flow of *kundalini* (*see* below)
- *bandhas* – body 'locks' that assist in controlling the flow of *prana*
- *pranayama* – purification of the *nadis* (the subtle channels of the body), through the control of the breath and vital inner pranic currents

As I have said, Patanjali does not specify any particular postures, saying only that the body must be kept motionless. I do not therefore intend to cover them here in any detail, although some traditional postures are dealt with in chapter 8. There are many excellent books which specialize in this subject alone. This chapter will deal with the *shatkarmas*, *mudras* and *bandhas* as well as the practices of fasting and yogic diet, which I feel are necessary in the purification of the mind and body. *Pranayama* will be covered in detail in the next chapter.

Kundalini (the coiled power) is the coiled-up energy present in all organic and inorganic matter. In the human being it lies dormant in the lower centre of consciousness at the base of the spine (*muladhara chakra*). Because *kundalini* is a spiralling power, it is symbolized as a coiled-up serpent.

When this vital force is awakened by the practice of such yogas as Kundalini, Laya, Kriya, Hatha, Raja or Bhakti, it forces a passage upwards through the chakras, via the *sushumna* canal (located within the spinal column, in the astral spine) from the *muladhara chakra* to the opening in the crown of the head (*sahasrara chakra*) and the yogi experiences higher levels of consciousness. When the *kundalini* reaches the *sahasrara chakra* the yogi attains supreme bliss.

PURIFICATION

Do you not know that your body is a temple of the Holy Spirit, who is in you, whom you have received from God? You are not your own; you were bought at a price. Therefore honour God with your body.

1 Corinthians 6:19–20

Blessed are the pure in heart, for they shall see God.

Matthew 5:8

Purity of heart is the fulfilment of non-attachment which those people achieve who are 'poor in spirit'. Non-attachment requires mental affirmation and self-effort, at least in the beginning of spiritual life. When non-attachment is perfected, it becomes purity of heart. Purity of heart is an effortless surrender of one's entire being into God's love. Purity of heart is achieved when one's feelings have been purged of all that is foreign to one's spiritual nature.

Sri Kriyananda, *Rays of the Same Light*, vol 3

The purpose of all spiritual practice (*sadhana*) is purification and inner transformation. As a result of purification and self-discipline, one experiences perfection and control of the body, mind and senses.

Purification is necessary to remove disease, toxins and impurities from the body. If the body is functioning in optimum health, the mind will also function properly.

Purification clears the mind of bad habits, inner resisting influences, restlessness, inertia, negative thoughts and emotions and negative attitudes. When your mind is clear and alert you can more easily develop an awareness of the presence of God.

Purification of the body and mind helps to awaken us from our identification with the sense of illusion, so that we can awaken to the reality of life, instead of the way it appears to us because of our conditioning and lack of understanding.

In reality we are perfect and self-complete, but until we purify the mind and clear all illusion and false understanding from it, the pure light of the soul within cannot be revealed or realized.

Affirmation

I am committed to the path of higher consciousness. I will engage in all useful disciplines to prepare myself for further purification and spiritual awakening. My body is the temple of spirit – the healing power within it heals, strengthens and perfects my mind and body. God's light and energy radiates through every tissue and cell of my body, making me whole and healthy.

I let go and let God, acknowledging that God is in charge. The presence of God is forever within me, restoring me to health and wholeness in mind, body and spirit. The divine intelligence within provides all the strength and guidance I need.

The *Shatkarmas*: Cleansing Techniques

Wrong diet and wrong living habits cause a build-up of toxins and impurities in the body tissues and block the body's channels. The aim of many of the Hatha Yoga techniques is to unblock the channels to revitalize and purify the body, preparing it for the higher spiritual practices. We need to take care of the body and keep it clean inside and outside, because it is a vehicle by which higher consciousness is attained. Revitalization of the body organism cannot be considered without being preceded by detoxification treatment. The yogi detoxifies the body, keeps it clean, healthy and vibrant with energy by practising the *shatkarmas* or the six purification techniques.

These techniques are both preventative and curative from a health point of view. They purify the body by removing impurities, excess mucus and toxins. They increase the body's resistance to disease and bring clarity and harmony to the mind. The *nadis* (subtle energy channels) are also purified by these techniques.

ASANA 117

The six main *shatkarmas* are as follows:

- *dhauti* – cleansing of the digestive tract
- *vasti* – colon cleansing
- *neti* – nasal cleansing
- *tratak* – steady gazing at an object or a particular point, without blinking
- *nauli* – intestinal cleansing
- *kapalabhati* – purification and vitalization of the frontal lobes of the brain.

Some of these *shatkarmas* have 'subdivisions' involving different techniques such as *jala neti, sutra neti, shankhaprakshalana, agni sara dhauti* and *danta dhauti*.

The *Hatha Yoga Pradipika* makes the point that those who wish to practise yoga who are of a flabby and phlegmatic constitution should first practise the six *shatkarmas*. This is particularly important before beginning the practice of intense *pranayama*. The reason for this is that there are three humours in the body: *kapha* (mucus), *pitta* (bile) and *vata* (wind). In Ayurveda (the science of life and healing), health is a state of dynamic equilibrium of the body elements – mucus, bile and wind. In Ayurveda they are called *tridoshas*. When any of the three *doshas* becomes excessively agitated or if there is an excess of one and a shortage of another, the healthy balance is lost and ailments or disease develop due to overheating or not enough heat in the body. So before starting *pranayama*, any imbalance in the *doshas* should be removed.

The practices cannot be effectively learned from a book. They are powerful, and one must be personally instructed how to perform them and how often, according to individual need. Please seek a qualified and experienced teacher in these practices, including the *shankhaprakshalana*, which cleans the complete digestive system from mouth to anus.

Dhauti

Wind purification
Benefits: to expel wind and gases from the stomach

Caution: to be practised under the guidance of an expert teacher.
Do not practice if you suffer from:
- stomach or intestinal ulcers
- hernia
- heart disease
- high blood pressure

or during menstruation

Method: To practise this *dhauti* one needs to swallow air to the stomach by closing the epiglottis. The yogi swallows small volumes of air to the stomach until the stomach is filled with air, then slowly expels the wind and gases from the stomach through the mouth.

Water purification

Kunjal kriya or vamana dhauti

Benefits: Cleans the upper digestive tract of mucus and excess acids. Good for digestive problems and headaches.

Caution: To be practised under the guidance of an expert teacher. Women should not practice during the menstrual cycle; this is to avoid any kind of hormonal or glandular imbalance within the body.

Practice time: early morning, before breakfast, once a week.

Method: Drink 4 pints (or 8 half-pint mugs) of lukewarm salt water (just below body temperature). Add 1 teaspoon of sea salt to 1 pint of water. Drink the water quickly one glass after another, then bend forward, contracting the stomach. At the same time rub the root of the tongue with the index and second fingers to induce vomiting of the water. After completing this practice, rest in *shavasana*, (relaxation pose) for 15–20 minutes.

Diet: Avoid spicy and acidic foods, including coffee, tea and chocolate.

Vastra dhauti (washing with a cloth)

Benefits: Good for excess bile and mucus problems, diseases of the stomach and spleen, gastritis, dyspepsia. It clears the bronchials and lungs, and is helpful in the treatment of asthma.

Caution: Do not practise without the guidance of an experienced teacher, and in full accordance with the instructions given. Females must *not* practise during menstrual cycle.

Practice time: Early morning on an empty stomach.

Method: You will need a finely woven muslin cotton cloth which is new and clean. The cloth should also be neatly trimmed so that there are no loose threads. The size of the cloth needs to be at least 1 metre and no more than 1½ metres in length. The width should be 2 inches (5 cm).

Sterilize the cloth in boiling water for a few minutes. Then dip it in lukewarm salt water and squeeze out the excess moisture.

Spread the cloth out, so that it does not fold as you use it. Either squat down on your heels or sit at a table on a chair to practise. Take one end of the cloth with both hands, and spread it over your tongue, then begin to swallow it by slowly sucking on it. If it catches in the throat and will not pass down, drink sips of warm water to lubricate the throat as you swallow the cloth little by little. The cloth tends to stick in the lowest point of the throat, but keep swallowing it and resist the urge to vomit. When the cloth has passed a little further down the oesophagus, there will be no problem. On the first day, swallow only 1 foot (30 cm), keep it there for a few seconds then take it out very slowly. On the second day, swallow a little more and so on until you have swallowed all the cloth except for 1 foot (30 cm) in order to remove it. Do not spend more than 30 minutes trying to swallow it. The cloth can be left in the stomach for 5–20 minutes but not longer. Then very slowly and carefully remove it.

Agni sara dhauti (fire purification)

Benefits: Stimulates liver, spleen, kidneys and pancreas. Good for constipation, tones the abdominal muscles. Creates heat at the navel centre (*manipura chakra*), purifying the *nadis* (subtle energy channels), and stimulating digestion.

Practice time: Daily on an empty stomach. The best time is early in the morning before breakfast. Good for awakening the *prana shakti* in preparation for meditation.

Method: Sit in a comfortable cross-legged posture. Inhale deeply, then exhale deeply, forcing as much air out of the lungs as possible. While holding the breath out, the diaphragm is automatically raised, and the abdominal muscles are pumped inward and outward in quick succession for as long as the breath can be held out without strain. Then inhale gently.

Start the practice with three rounds and increase gradually to ten, so that you are practising ten rounds of 20 daily.

Danta dhauti (cleaning of the tongue, teeth, throat, ears, eyes and forehead)

The mouth is the gate-keeper of the digestive system and the tongue functions as an organ of elimination. When you get up in the morning, you will probably find when you look in the mirror that your tongue is coated with a white mucus, composed of bacteria and dead cells (leucocytes). These toxins need to be expelled to keep the mouth sweet and clean.

Tongue: To clean the tongue, join your index, middle and ring fingers together and insert them into your mouth. Rub the root of the tongue with your fingers and water. Wash your fingers and rinse your mouth out and repeat the process several times until the coated tongue becomes a healthy, pink colour. Rubbing the root of the tongue will also cause a gagging reflex, which will clear out any excess mucus.

The amount of mucus on the tongue indicates the state of the digestive system. With a clean, pink tongue, one is able to absorb *prana* from food more effectively.

One can also clean the tongue with a toothbrush, by lightly brushing the top surface with water.

Teeth: If the mouth is kept unclean and food particles are allowed to stick in the crevices of the teeth (combining with bacteria to produce an acid), decay sets in and diseases of the gums such as pyorrhoea and gingivitis take a hold, causing pain and suffering. Many germs and bacteria breed in an unclean mouth. To give you an idea of the amount of bacteria living around the gums and teeth, an estimate by modern counting methods yielded approximately 5 million cocci bacteria per milligram of scrapings from the gum cleft.

Proper cleaning of the teeth and gums along with proper nutrition is important for healthy teeth and gums.

The ideal toothbrush to use is one with a head less than 1 inch long, with its bristles arranged in a straight line. Nylon bristles that are soft to medium with smooth, rounded ends will not scratch the tooth enamel or tender gums.

There are a number of natural toothpastes on the market containing plant and herb oils and extracts. There are two that I particularly recommend.

- Vicco Vajradanti herbal ayurvedic toothpaste from India. It contains 18 herbs and bark extracts.
- Parodontax, a medicinal toothpaste against periodontitis and dental caries. Made by Madaus in Germany, it contains various plant and herb extracts: myrrh (strengthens tissue); ratanhia (astringes the gums); sage (deodorizes); chamomile (inhibits inflammation); echinacea (stimulates resistance, reinforcing tissue defences). This toothpaste also includes sodium bicarbonate in a stabilized form, which neutralizes the acids which attack the enamel of the teeth.

Brush the biting surfaces and the surfaces away from the gum a few times. Then gently insert the toothbrush bristles as far as possible at a 45-degree angle within the crevice where the teeth meet the gums. Now wiggle the brush back and forth, using short strokes.

To brush the front teeth, hold the brush vertically with the bristles inserted into the gum crevice. Then rinse the mouth out with water and gargle.

Use dental floss once or twice a day to clean between the teeth, where a brush cannot reach. Remember to floss methodically from the last tooth, upper or lower, and continue from tooth to tooth until all the crevices between the teeth are flossed. Then rinse the mouth out with water.

Remember to change your toothbrush as soon as it begins to go out of shape.

Stick to a balanced wholefood/vegetarian diet, avoiding sugar-laden foods that cling to the teeth and gums. A raw diet is good, because fibrous foods such as apples, carrots and celery stimulate a greater flow of saliva, which helps to remove debris from the mouth.

In India it is a custom to chew a few neem leaves to keep the mouth sweet and clean. Neem leaves act as a powerful germicide.

Throat: Mouthwashes and gargles with salt water help to keep the throat clean and free from infection.

Sage is a good gargle for sore throats. Use one teaspoonful of sage to one cup of boiling water. Steep for several minutes and strain. Gargle and sip morning and evening as required.

Ears: Wet the middle finger and clean the opening of the ear. If the ear is blocked with wax, it can be softened by pressing firmly but gently behind the ear, in front of the ear, and then by gently pulling the ear lobe up and down. This stimulates ear circulation and can be repeated daily.

Syringing of the ears can be harmful, so use a cotton bud and massage the ear first to remove wax that has hardened.

On no account try to probe into the ear with wires, sticks etc, as the tissues of the ear are very delicate.

Eyes: Bathe the eyes with tepid saline water. Another way is to fill a bowl or basin with cold water, hold your breath and plunge your face in with eyes open, and move the eyeballs upwards, downwards and circularly. Then gently pat the skin area around the eyes with a dry towel.

You can also clean your eyes by scooping clean cold water up into the palms of your hands and splashing it over the face to flush the eyes.

Forehead: Rub the depression between the forehead and the nose with the thumb of the right hand. This purifies the nervous system and clairvoyance is induced.

Vasti

There are two techniques of *vasti*, *sthala vasti* or *vata vasti*, which cleans the colon by sucking air into the body, and *jala vasti*, whereby one sucks water into the anus.

Benefits: Vasti completely washes the bowel and removes excess bacteria, old stool, threadworms and heat from the lower intestines. It is good for digestive disorders, constipation and urinary problems and strengthens the abdominal muscles. The *Hatha Yoga Pradipika* says:

> *By practising* jala vasti *the appetite increases, the body glows, excess* doshas *are destroyed and the* dhatu, *senses and mind are purified.*
>
> 2:28

It also improves and purifies the blood supply, controls nervous diarrhoea and pushes apana vayu upward.

Caution: Vasti should *not* be practised by anyone with a fever, ulcers, haemorrhoids, high blood pressure, hernia or any serious digestive ailments. Women should *not* practise during the menstrual cycle.

Practice time: If you have normal bowel movements, once a week; if you have loose bowels, twice a month; if you have constipation, twice a week.

Method: The practice of *vasti* induces a great flow of pranic energy. It stimulates the pranic energy, making one feel very active and dynamic afterwards. However, this practice also removes heat and energy from the physical body. The water absorbs the heat of the body and draws it out when the water gushes out. It is important that one practices *vasti* in a warm room or outside in warm, dry weather. If the body loses heat and is unable to regain it, it may suffer from constipation.

Squat in a tub or bath of lukewarm water up to the level of the navel. Take a small tube (rubber catheter) about 6 inches (15 cm) long and $1/2$ inch (10–12 mm) wide. Make sure it has been sterilized first. Mark the middle of the tube with string or tape and lubricate one end with pure vegetable oil. Gently insert the tube about 3 inches into the rectum, then squat, exhale and practise *nauli kriya* (rolling and isolation of the abdominal rectus muscles – see pages 141–2), which creates a vacuum, drawing the water into the large intestine. If the water is not sucked up through the tube into the bowel, then practise *madhyama nauli* and hold; if this does not work, then practise *vama* or *dakshia nauli*. When you can no longer hold your breath out (*kumbhaka*), remove the tube without exhaling. Then stand up and exhale slowly through the nose. When you do this it is advisable to squat over the toilet because stool in the lower intestine will also come out.

After the practice, lie in *shavasana* (relaxation pose) on a blanket and slowly assume *pashinee mudra* (the folded *mudra* -- see pages 158–9). This releases air from the bowel and induces a bowel action if there is any water remaining. Come out of the position slowly and rest for one hour before beginning your daily activities.

Shankhaprakshalana or *Varisara Dhauti*

Shank means conch shell, which has convolutions resembling the intestines and *prakshalana* means 'to wash thoroughly'.

This practice is the most comprehensive of the Hatha Yoga cleansing processes. It gives the most thorough and complete cleansing of the entire length of the digestive and eliminative system from mouth to rectum. It requires no apparatus or expense and it is simple and safe under the supervision of an expert teacher who is experienced in this practice.

The cleansing process is a lengthy one, which can take about four or five hours to complete. It completely removes all the hardened faeces that have stuck to the walls of the colon and which do not pass out with regular bowel movements, which may include post-putrefactive matter that began to accumulate shortly after birth! Diet alone will not remove these old faeces that may have built up in pockets, coating the entire length of the colon and small intestines. It thus requires a special technique that dissolves the glue which binds them to the body. The longer the material remains in the colon, the more moisture is absorbed from it and the more dry and compressed it becomes.

Can you imagine your colon being packed with a lifetime's accumulation of old black and grey hardened faeces! These can deform the shape and provide a breeding ground for harmful bacteria. These bacteria and toxins from the decaying process travel into the bloodstream to all parts of the body, causing disease.

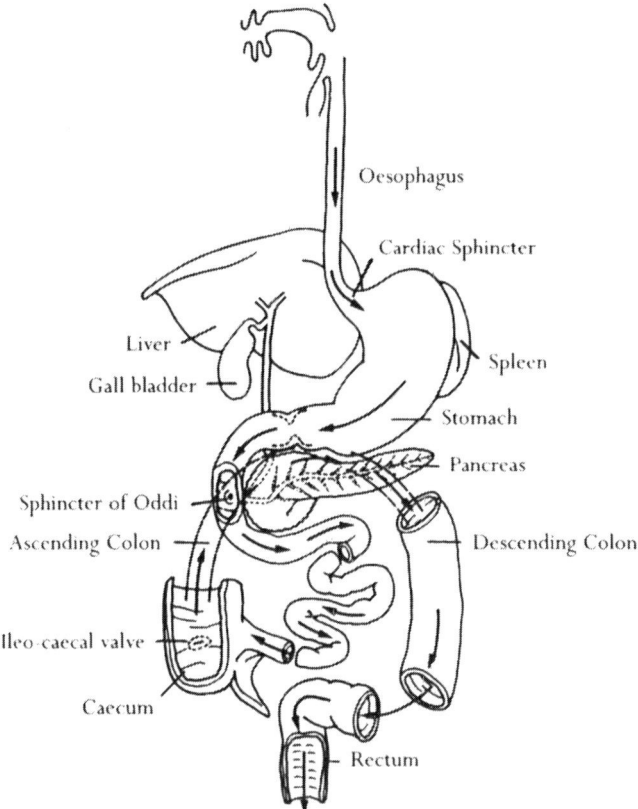

Figure 12 *The digestive system – showing the flow of warm salt water in the practice of shankhaprakshalana*

Benefits: This practice improves digestion and is recommended for those who suffer from chronic constipation, acidity, gas and digestive upset. It is good for the kidneys and urinary system.

It purifies the *nadis* (subtle energy channels) and makes the body feel light. It cleans both physically and mentally by removing and releasing blocks in the mind and body systems.

The treatment of psychosomatic illnesses such as asthma, migraines and allergies have had a good success in cure, using *shankhaprakshalana* as a part of the therapy.

Caution: Do not practise without the expert guidance of an experienced teacher. It is also better to practise with a few other people to help enthusiasm and to help you to be positive and cheerful. Be positive and lighthearted, as it can be quite a tiring and lengthy process to practise, especially the first time. Women should *not* practise during the menstrual cycle.

Keep warm throughout the practice.

Practice time: Early in the morning on an empty stomach; Practise every six months – the best times are the beginning of spring and autumn.

Eat lightly the day before you practise (fruit and salad would be ideal). Or from noon onwards you could fast, drinking only pure fruit juice or pure water. On the morning before the practice commences completely fast from food and drink. The reason for eating lightly or fasting the day before is so that you will not have so much waste to eliminate from the body on the day of the practice.

Preparation: Prepare about two or three gallons of very warm salt water. Add one teaspoon of salt to each pint of water.

- Salt water leaves the stomach faster than ordinary water.
- Salt helps to dissolve the contents of the intestines so that elimination of wastes and impurities is made easier.
- Salt is not absorbed into the blood, whereas amino acids and sugar are.
- The correct quantity of salt ensures that the water drunk is not excreted through the kidneys, but remains mostly in the intestines and is evacuated through the rectum.
- Osmotic pressure (salt/water ratio) remains the same on both sides of the intestinal wall, so that the body's normal salt and liquid concentration is not disturbed.

Method: Using a half-pint mug or glass, drink two glasses of the salt water quickly. Then practice the following *asanas* in the order shown. In order to prevent nausea, breathe deeply while practising them.

1 *Tadasana:* Stand with your feet about 6 inches apart, interlock the fingers and turn the palms upwards, stretching your arms above your

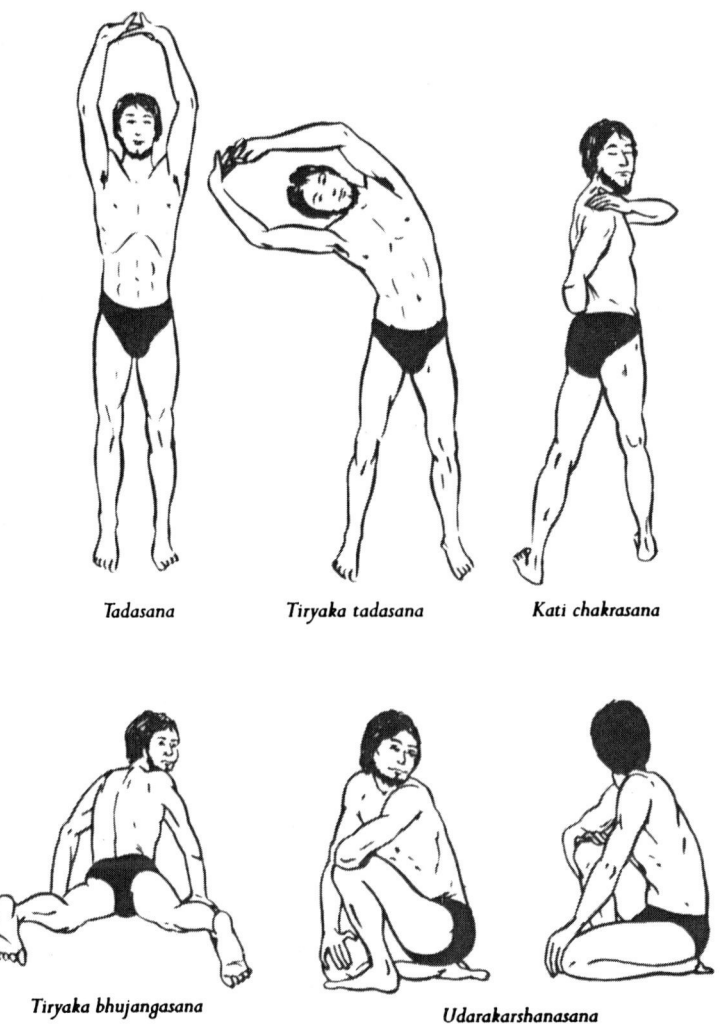

Figure 13 Shankaprakshalana – *practise these five asanas eight times each*

head. Rise up onto your toes and completely stretch your whole body. Then slowly relax. Practise eight times.
2. *Tiryaka tadasana:* Stand with your feet about 2½ feet apart. Interlock your fingers and turn your palms upwards, stretching your arms above your head, balancing on your toes. Then bend from the waist to the right side and then to the left. Practise eight times to each side.
3. *Kati chakrasana* (waist rotating pose): With your feet 2½ feet apart, rotate your body from the waist upwards so that your arms swing loosely out from your body. Twisting to the right, look as far back as you can over your right shoulder, with the left hand resting on the right shoulder. The left arm is bent at the elbow and swings round to touch the lower back. Repeat on the other side. Practise eight times.
4. *Tiryaka bhujangasana* (twisting cobra pose): Lie on your stomach with your palms flat on the floor beneath your shoulders. Spread your legs 2½ feet apart and raise your trunk off the floor by straightening your arms. Then twist your head to the right and look back at your heels; then twist to the left and look back. Practise eight times to each side.
5. *Udarakarshanasana* (stomach squeezing pose): Squat down with your feet apart, hands on knees. Bring your body's weight to the ball of your left foot by sitting on your left heel. At the same time bring your left knee down to meet your right foot. Twist your upper body to the right and look over your right shoulder. With your right hand, press your knee and thigh in against your stomach and abdomen. Practise eight times to the right and the left.

Immediately after these five *asanas*, drink another two glasses of warm salt water, then repeat the five *asanas* eight times each again. Drink another two glasses and repeat the *asanas* until six glasses have been drunk. Then go to the toilet. Even if you have no urge to go, sit on the toilet.

Gradually, as you keep drinking the water, the pressure will build up inside. Try to keep this pressure up, then the water will come out quickly.

Continue this process of drinking water, practising the five *asanas* and going to the toilet until a clear water is passed through the anus

(90 per cent of the water under pressure will be released through the anus), only slightly coloured by bile. Then stop.

At the beginning of this practice you will pass fairly solid stools; they will break up more and more as the practice goes on, until the stools become very watery. Finally water will be passed through the anus.

Constantly going to the toilet, with salt water pouring through your anus, can make your anus feel a bit sore, so when you have finished, lubricate the area with some pure vegetable oil.

It may take over 20 glasses of water to clean your digestive/ eliminative system out – it varies with each individual. It takes considerably less water for those yogis who have practised *shankhaprakshalana* a few times before.

If you smoke and are full of toxins through eating meat and junk food, and you practise *shankhaprakshalana* for the very first time, you may feel an urge to vomit. If so, then vomit, but afterwards drink as much water as was vomited.

To help activate the flow and pressure of water through the intestines, squat down with the soles of your feet flat on the floor and your knees pressed against your abdomen, and rest your arms on your knees. One can also practise additional *asanas* like *dhanurasana* (the bow), *chakrasana* (the wheel) or *pavanamuktasana* (gas- and wind-eliminating pose) (see figure 14) to help the water to flow through the body.

Pavanamuktasana (gas- and wind-eliminating pose)

Method:
1 Lie down on your back.
2 Inhale deeply as you bend your left knee towards your chest. Your hands should be locked together and clasped tightly around the knee, pulling your knee down to squeeze your thigh against your abdomen. Bring your forehead to your knee.
3 Hold your breath in this pose.
4 Exhale deeply while lowering your leg and your head.
5 Repeat with right leg; then with both legs together. The whole process can be repeated three to five times. Then completely relax.

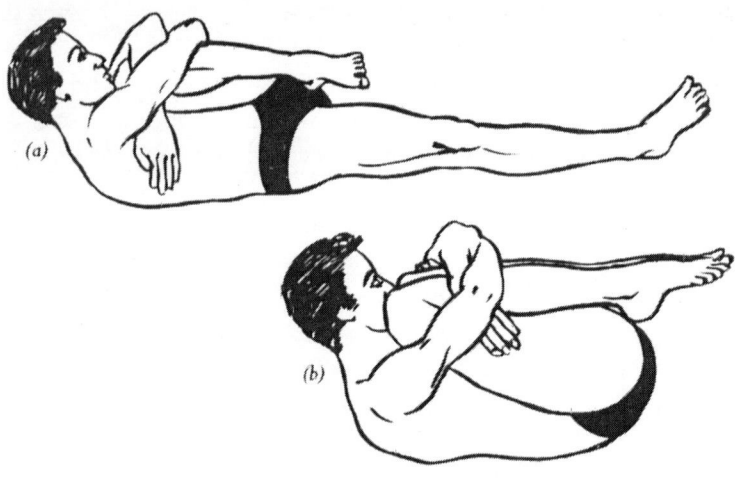

Figure 14 Pavanamuktasana *(gas- and wind-eliminating pose)*

Dhanurasana (the bow)

Method:
1 Lie down on your front, with your forehead resting on the floor.
2 Bend your knees and grasp your ankles with your hands. Allow your knees to be slightly apart.
3 Inhale and raise your head, chest and thighs off the ground as high as possible; so that your body is resting on your abdomen.
4 Hold your breath for three deep breaths while holding the pose.
5 Exhale as you lower your body down and relax.
6 Repeat twice more. Try 'rocking' backwards and forwards in the final pose to massage the abdomen.

Benefits: This is an excellent *asana* to massage and invigorate all the internal organs. Tones up the abdominal muscles. Regulates the pancreas, liver and spleen. Gives flexibility to the spine. Good for people who have diabetes.

Caution: This posture should not be practised by pregnant women.

Chakrasana (the wheel)

Method:
1 Lie down on your back with your knees bent, and pull your feet close to your buttocks.
2 Place your hands beside your ears, palms flat on the floor with your fingers pointing towards the shoulders.
3 With your feet flat on the floor, raise your hips as high as possible. Inhale and slowly raise your body up, by pushing with your hands and feet. Arch your back and neck, and rest the crown of your head on the floor between your hands. *Exhale.* In this stage the elbows are still bent.
4 Inhale as you straighten your elbows and push up with your hands and feet, arching your hips and chest as high as comfortable. Breathe deeply while holding the pose.
5 Exhale and slowly lower your body to the floor.

Benefits: Invigorates and tones the whole body. Gives flexibility to the spine. Strengthens the arms and legs. Massages the abdominal organs and muscles. Removes sluggishness of the liver and gastro-intestinal disorders.

Caution: Not to be practised by people with hernia, peptic ulcers or intestinal tuberculosis.

After practising *shankhaprakshalana* go on to practise *kunjal kriya* (see page 118), then *jala neti* (see pages 135–7).

On completion of these practices lie down in a quiet room and rest in *shavasana* (relaxation pose – see page 132) for 45 minutes to an hour. Relax completely, but do not sleep.

After resting it is necessary to eat a specially prepared meal (do not let more than one hour elapse before eating), consisting of polished boiled rice (whole brown rice is difficult to digest after doing this practice), pulse or lentils and ghee (clarified butter). This mixture in India is called *kicheri*.

The recipe is as follows. Take three parts rice to one part lentils. One cupful of this dry mixture will easily suffice one person after cooking. While it is cooking in water, add a tiny quantity of ground

Shavasana (relaxation pose or corpse pose)

Method: In a warm but well-ventilated room lie down on a mat with a blanket covering your body to keep warm. Your body should be straight but relaxed, with your feet slightly apart, your arms slightly away from the body, palms upwards. Close your eyes and completely relax your whole body. Breathe deeply for a few minutes, being aware of each breath as it flows in and flows out. Remain aware of the breath and how the mind is aware of the breath.

Now bring your awareness to your body. Rotate your consciousness through each part of the body. Begin by bringing your awareness to your feet and mentally repeat: 'I am aware of my feet, I let go of all tension and relax them.' Repeat the same process as you bring your awareness to each body part. Continue in this order:

1 feet
2 shins
3 kneecaps
4 thighs
5 abdomen (navel to pubic bone)
6 solar plexus (navel to breastbone)
7 upper chest
8 spine
9 hands
10 forearms
11 upper arms
12 throat
13 back of the head
14 jaw, facial muscles
15 nose, eyes, ears
16 scalp, crown of head

After rotating the consciousness through your body, become *aware* of your breath — breathe consciously and be aware of the sense of feeling in your body. Feel the weight of your body lying on the floor. Begin to slowly move your fingers and toes. Roll your head gently from side to side.

Slowly stretch your arms behind your body as you breathe in, lengthening the whole body. Yawn if you need to, breathe out and relax. Roll over on to your side and slowly sit up, opening your eyes.

turmeric root (powdered), sufficient to make the mix appear yellow. When the grain is well cooked and the consistency is like thin porridge, serve a large plateful with a teaspoon of ghee mixed into it. This is to lubricate the intestines, because the mucous membrane of the alimentary canal has been somewhat stripped by the practice of *shankhaprakshalana*. If, after one plateful, you can eat more, then do, because the main purpose of the meal is to provide packing, lubrication and relining of the alimentary canal. Eat as much as you want, but the food must be warm, not too hot or cold. Another *kicheri* meal may be taken in the evening at least three hours before sleep.

Spend the rest of the day in a relaxed, peaceful atmosphere, but do not sleep until the evening. Be aware of any changes which take place physically, mentally and emotionally within you. Many people experience wonderful peace of mind, increased energy and vitality after practising *shankhaprakshalana*. This practice certainly removes impurities both from the body and the mind (mental blocks).

For the next ten days there are certain dietary restrictions that one must follow: *no* meat, fish, eggs, tea, coffee, chocolate, alcohol, tobacco, drugs, all forms of sugar, sweets, strong spices, garlic, onions, leeks, raw vegetables and all dairy produce.

Smoking should definitely be avoided. If you are trying to stop smoking, then this is a very good practice, because your increased sensitivity will help you to be more aware of the unpleasant aspects of filling your lungs with a pollutant.

For the next 30 days avoid meat, fish or eggs. For the next ten days your diet should consist mainly of cooked whole grains (millet, rice, wholewheat, oats, etc), beans and pulses and cooked vegetables (steam the vegetables lightly). Use a pure vegetable oil (grapeseed, sunflower or safflower).

After the ten-day cooked food diet you can begin to add fresh fruits, raw vegetables and a little dairy produce, as well as seeds and nuts for a well-balanced vegetarian/wholefood diet.

After purifying your body by means of *shankhaprakshalana*, do not fall back into your old habits. Resolve always to remain healthy, functional and radiantly alive with vitality and energy. Make the following affirmation.

> My body is the temple of the spirit and radiates the light and energy of God through every system and body cell. I align my thoughts with the divine intelligence within me, and achieve freedom from all that would block the flow of healing energy in and through me. Abundant energy is mine. God is glorified through my physical form.

To stop the build-up of faeces again, it is advisable to reduce the mucus-forming foods in your diet. Each of us has the ability to create health or disease. We are responsible for our own health. If our bodies are to function optimally in good health, then we need to remove those foods that upset our body chemistry and eat wholesome, natural vegetarian foods that create good health and balance in the physical body. The mucus-forming foods are:

- dairy products (especially those derived from cow's milk – goat's milk is less mucus-forming)
- meat, fish and eggs
- sugar and sugar products
- salt
- white flour and flour products
- gas-ripened bananas

Vegetables and fruits (especially when eaten raw) are non-mucus forming.

There is a short form of the cleansing technique that you practise by yourself, called *laghoo shankhaprakshalana*.

Practice time: Early morning on an empty stomach, once a week.

Method: Drink two glasses of warm salt water. Perform the five *asanas* eight times each, then sit on the toilet. Complete this cycle twice more. The complete cycle will take eight glasses of salt water and three complete rounds of the five asanas.

Then rest in *shavasana* (relaxation pose) for 20–30 minutes. Wait at least 30 minutes before eating breakfast. There is no special diet to follow.

Of course with the short cleansing, it is unlikely that you will completely cleanse the system, but this short wash is definitely recommended for people who may be suffering from constipation (usually caused by stress, tension and poor nutrition).

Note: Shankhaprakshalana should not be seen as the ultimate treatment for all diseases of the digestive system, but together with the practice of *asanas, pranayama,* meditation, proper rest, proper exercise and eating a balanced vegetarian/wholefood diet, it will promote a free flow of body energies and help to enhance homoeostasis (when the body chemistry is in balance).

Neti

When we breathe in air we also breathe in bacteria, pollen and dust. To prevent this foreign matter from entering the lungs, nature has designed a perfect filtering system.

The path that the air follows is determined by the shape of the nasal cavity inside the nose. The nasal cavity has three turbinates, whose function is to circulate the air as it enters the nose so that the stream of air passes over a great surface. These turbinates have a great effect on the moisture content and temperature of the entering air. As the air enters it passes over the warm, moist turbinates, drawing to it humidity and heat. When we breathe out, the air passes over the turbinates which have just been cooled and dried by the incoming air and rewarms and moistens them, preventing loss of heat and moisture from the body.

The inside of the nose is lined with a covering, called a mucous membrane, which secretes mucus. In the mucous membranes and sinuses are found numerous tiny hairlike structures, called cilia, which all quiver in the same direction. A layer of mucus covers the cilia and traps bacteria, viruses, dust and pollen, carrying them down the nose, throat and eventually into the intestinal tract where the digestive enzymes dissolve both the mucus and the bacteria.

Sometimes the ciliary movement is affected if the mucus is too thick or viscous and dries out easily, becoming crusted and hard. It is at this stage that bacteria begins to invade. It can also be a problem if the mucus is too runny, for it drips down around the cilia and reduces their effectiveness in keeping the mucus together. Again, infection can occur.

The sinuses are also lined with mucous membrane and can secrete mucus, although their function is to remain hollow.

The mucus secretions produced in the sinuses are continually being swept into the nose by the ciliated surface of the respiratory membranes. If the tiny passageways that lead down into the nasal cavity are blocked then inflammation occurs, causing sinusitis and sinus headache.

Jala neti (nasal cleaning with water)

Benefits: The practice of *jala neti* helps in preventing and eliminating sinusitis and sinus headaches by promoting drainage of the sinuses, preventing stasis of mucus and keeping them clean and functional. It maintains healthy secretory and drainage mechanisms of the entire ear (including the eustachian tubes in the nasopharynx), nose and throat area. This helps to ward off colds, coughs, catarrh, hay fever and tonsillitis. *Jala neti* also strengthens the eyes, because there is stimulation of the blood vessels of the eyes and nose. It exerts a relaxing and irrigating effect upon the eyes by stimulating the tear ducts and glands.

On an emotional level, it releases tensions and is beneficial in depression, anxiety, and hysteria.

This practice also promotes a balance between the left and right nostrils, balancing the right and left hemispheres of the brain and the entire central nervous system. It gives mental clarity and helps in creating a balanced flow of *prana* in the three *nadis: ida*, *pingala* and *sushumna*.

Caution: Seek the guidance of a qualified teacher who can instruct you correctly and safely in this practice. Do not practise in the evening before going to bed, because water may remain in the nostril and cause sinusitis or a cold. Those suffering from chronic haemorrhage should not attempt *neti*.

Practice time: Neti can be practised every day if you are suffering from colds, catarrh, sinusitis, headaches, eyestrain or eye infections, otherwise it is best to practise only twice a week.

Method: Take a small pot with an extended spout that fits comfortably into the entrance of the nostril. You can buy *neti* pots that are specifically designed for this purpose. The pot needs to hold at least $\frac{1}{2}$ pint of water.

Fill the pot with lukewarm salt water, one teaspoon of salt to one pint of water. Too little salt will create pain, while too much will cause a burning sensation.

Now stand with your legs apart and lean forward over a bath or sink if you are inside a building. Outside you can stand in the garden. Keep the whole body relaxed. Take the pot of salt water and hold the spout to one nostril, while tilting the head slightly forward and to the side. Breathe through your mouth. Let the water run in one nostril and pass out through the other. If the head is tilted properly, the water will easily flow down and out of the lower nostril. Now with the head centred again blow the nose to clear the nostril of water. Then repeat the process again using the other nostril.

If one nostril seems to be blocked before you practise then begin your practice by pouring the water into the nostril through which you are breathing freely. The nostril which is open provides an easier entry for the water within the nasal passage, and that water, once it enters, is able to force its way out through the other nostril much more easily.

You can also pour the salt water through one nostril, closing the other nostril with the thumb. Then raising the head you allow the water to flow down to the throat and out of the mouth.

After practising *jala neti* you may find that you still have some water left in your nasal passages, so to drain it out, stand with your feet 2 feet apart and bend forward from the waist, so that the head is lower than the waist. Remain like this for a minute or two, to allow excess water to trickle down into the nostrils. Then closing one nostril with the thumb, blow the air out with the water in short, sharp bursts, still keeping the head lower than the waist. Repeat with the other nostril.

Afterwards sit in *vajrasana* (kneeling on your heels) and practise a few rounds of *bhastrika pranayama* (see chapter 5) and *kapalabhati* (see pages 142–4), first through one nostril, closing the other with the thumb, then through the other. This will dry the nose and generate heat in the nostrils.

Vajrasana (the thunderbolt pose)

Method: Kneel down and sit on your heels, with your feet stretched back. Keep your knees together and your heels apart. Cross your left big toe over your right big toe.

Buttocks should sit on the insides of feet with heels at the sides of hips.

Place your hands on your knees, palms downward. Sit for as long as comfortable, breathing normally and relaxed. To improve your digestive system sit for at least 5 minutes in this pose.

Benefits: Increases the efficiency of the entire digestive system. Strengthens the pelvic muscles; reduces blood flow to the genitals and massages the nerve fibres which feed them.

Sutra neti (nasal cleaning with string)

Benefits: This practice is beneficial for the eyes, clearing the nasal passageways and strengthening the mucous membranes.

The soft cotton string will absorb and clean various foreign particles accumulated in the nasal passages.

Caution: Seek the guidance of a qualified teacher who can instruct you carefully and safely in this practice. Do not practise *sutra neti* if you have frequent nose bleeds or lesions inside the nose. If you have a deviated septum, use a thin string first, then gradually increase its thickness.

Practice time: May be practised twice a week.

Method: The method of *sutra neti* is practised by passing a length of thread through the nose.

Traditionally the thread used by yogis in India is specially prepared. It is made of cotton, tightly wound together and then wiped with melted beeswax (so that it is hard enough to push through the nasal cavity). However, it is more convenient to use a thin rubber catheter which can be bought from a surgical shop.

The string or catheter must be sterilized in boiling water and then lubricated with ghee (traditionally), or vegetable oil, before inserting it into the nose. Another way is to wet the string or catheter in warm salt water before insertion into the nose.

Before you start the *sutra neti* practice, it is a good idea to practise *jala neti* first to make sure the nostrils are clear. Then squat or sit and

ASANA 139

tilt the head slightly back, and insert the thread or catheter gently into one nostril, pushing it gently so that it passes slowly down into the throat. When it reaches the back of the throat (look in a mirror), insert the first two fingers into the mouth and pull the thread out through the mouth, leaving a few inches of thread hanging out of the nose. Slowly and gently pull the thread backwards and forwards 30 times. Remove it slowly and repeat the same process with the other nostril.

When you have finished, practice *pranayama*.

Nauli

The Sanskrit word *nala* or *nali*, means a tubular vessel, vein or nerve of the body, a reed or a hollow stalk. It is also the Sanskrit word for the rectus abdomini. It is also interesting to note that the Sanskrit word *nau* means 'ship', for when *nauli* is perfected, the abdominal muscles seem to flow or roll like the rolling waves of the ocean. The muscles create the same wave-like motion as that produced by a ship.

Nauli is the practice of contracting and isolating the rectus abdominal muscles. These two long vertical muscles, situated in front of the abdomen, originate at the pubic bone and are attached to the cartilages of the fifth, sixth and seventh ribs above. Though these are the muscles you are manipulating in *nauli*, the external oblique, internal oblique and transversalis muscles are also utilized.

At first *nauli* is practised with the hands just above the knees, with the body leaning forward. Once this is perfected you can practise in the more erect position, with the hands placed on the upper thighs.

Benefits: The ancient yogi Swatmarama, author of the *Hatha Yoga Pradipika*, informs us that *nauli* is the most important of all the Hatha Yoga practices. It kindles the digestive fire, removing sluggish digestion.

Nauli prevents dyspepsia and constipation. It strengthens, tones and invigorates the abdominal muscles and removes sluggishness from the stomach, intestines and liver. It is a corrective for the liver, spleen, pancreas and kidneys. *Nauli* balances the endocrine system and helps control the production of sex hormones.

It increases heat in the navel area, which aids digestion, elimination and blood circulation. It is also good for alleviating sexual and urinary

Madhyama nauli (central contraction)

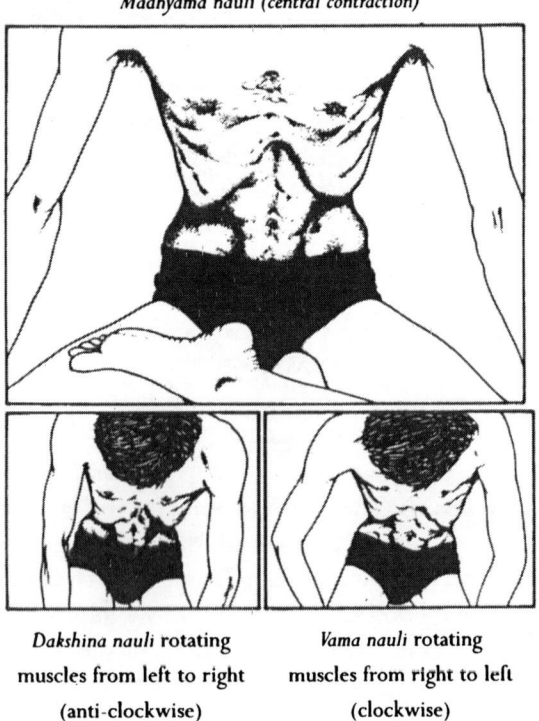

| *Dakshina nauli* rotating muscles from left to right (anti-clockwise) | *Vama nauli* rotating muscles from right to left (clockwise) |

Figure 15 *Nauli kriya*

disorders, lack of energy and hormonal imbalances. The nerve plexuses and their fine terminals in the pelvic region are stimulated.

Caution: Seek the guidance of a qualified teacher who can instruct you carefully and safely in this practice. First master *uddiyana bandha* (see below) before practising *nauli*, as it takes time to bring the abdominal muscles under control.

    Nauli should not be performed by those suffering from or suspected of abdominal tuberculosis or chronic colitis, heart disease, high blood pressure, hernia, peptic or duodenal ulcer or gallstones. It is contra-indicated in chronic appendicitis. Pregnant women should not practise it, but it is highly recommended after childbirth to strengthen the abdominal and pelvic muscles. Boys and girls of a pre-pubertal age should not perform this exercise. Avoid during menstruation.

Practice time: Daily, early in the morning on an empty stomach (at least five to six hours after meals).

If you feel any pain in the abdomen during *nauli* you should immediately stop the practice and resume when the pain subsides.

Method for uddiyana bandha: Stand with your feet about 2 feet apart with your knees slightly bent. Place your hands firmly on your thighs just above the knees, with the thumbs on the inside of your thighs and fingers touching the outside. Bend your trunk slightly forward and keep your head up. Breathe in deeply through your nose and empty your lungs by exhaling quickly through your mouth, slightly pursing your lips as you do so. Apply the *jalandhara bandha* (chin lock) (see page 154–5) while holding the breath out. This will cause the diaphragm to rise naturally to the thoracic cavity. Now pull the intestines and navel up and back towards the spine. Hold this position for as long as you can comfortably hold your breath out. Finally, release *uddiyana bandha* first, then *jalandhara bandha*. Raise the head and slowly inhale through the nose as you stand up straight and relax. Take a few breaths before starting the next round. Repeat three or four times.

Method for nauli:
1 As in *uddiyana bandha*, stand in the same position. Practise *uddiyana* with the diaphragm raised, pulling the intestines and navel up and back.

    While maintaining *uddiyana*, press your palms just above your knees, and give a forward and slightly downward thrust to the abdominal portion between the umbilicus and the pubic bone. The push at this region contracts the rectus muscles keeping the other muscles of the abdomen in a relaxed condition. The equal pressure on both knees further helps one to achieve the perfect isolation of both the abdominal rectus muscles and to make them stand side by side in the centre. This is known as *madhyama nauli* (the central aspect of *nauli*).

    I would advise that you practise before a mirror to watch what progress you are making and whether you are performing the technique correctly. The whole of the abdomen must not be contracted; only the rectus muscles are to be isolated. This is but the first part of the whole exercise of isolation. You can only proceed to the other part when this has been thoroughly mastered.

2   The next part consists in isolating each rectus muscle separately and rolling them alternately in a wave-like movement.

   While maintaining the central isolation of the rectus muscles, bend forward. If the right rectus is to be isolated lean a little more on the right side, keeping the left side of the abdomen relaxed. The pressure just above the right knee is increased, while simultaneously the pressure on the left thigh is removed. In this way one is able to contract and roll the rectus muscle to the extreme right side, while the left rectus remains relaxed. This isolation of the right rectus muscle is called *dakshina nauli*.

   The same technique applies to the left rectus by leaning on the left thigh and simultaneously applying more pressure just above the left knee, making the left rectus muscle isolated and rolled off to the extreme left side. The isolation of the left rectus muscle is known as *vama nauli*.

3   When the recti have been brought under perfect control singly, one is ready to roll them from side to side. This is achieved by performing *vama nauli* and then rolling the muscles to the right and back to the left. The rotation of the rectus muscle is continued in a clockwise direction (known as churning). Start by practising three times consecutively, then release. Practise *dakshina nauli* (isolation of right rectus) in the same way, rotating the muscles anti-clockwise. When this churning is perfected, practise it three times with *vama nauli* (left rectus), then three times with *dakshina nauli* and release. When this is perfected you can increase from three to seven rounds, taking a few normal breaths with the body relaxed in between each round if necessary. The whole sequence of rotation should be practised without any discomfort, pain or strain at any stage.

Kapalabhati

In Sanskrit, *kapala* means 'skull' and *bhati* means 'shine', 'light' or 'splendour'. *Kapalabhati* is a *pranayama* technique which invigorates the entire brain and awakens the dormant centres which are responsible for subtle perception.

   This purificatory process involves the breathing apparatus, the nasal passages and the sinuses in the skull that are cleansed effectively. It is a similar practice to *bhastrika pranayama* (*see* chapter 5), except that exhalation is emphasized and inhalation is the result of forcing the air out.

The *Gheranda Samhita*, an ancient yogic text, mentions three varieties of *kapalabhati* whose main characteristic is cleansing the nasal passages of the skull: *vatakrama, vyutkrama* and *sheetkrama*. Here we are mainly concerned with *vatakrama kapalabhati*, which involves the breath without using water. *Vyutkrama* is similar to *jala neti*. Warm salt water is scooped up in the palm of the hand and then it is sniffed up into the nostrils and expelled out through the mouth, and *sheetkrama* is the reverse: one takes a mouthful of warm salty water, but instead of swallowing it, one expels it through the nose.

Benefits: Kapalabhati stimulates the nerves. In turn they activate the *nadis*, which then activate the *pranas*. The *pranas* then gravitate towards the area where the action is taking place in the frontal lobes of the brain. This brings an awakening to the spiritual eye (*ajna chakra*).

Kapalabhati purifies the respiratory passage, keeping it clear from impurities and mucus. It purifies the *nadis* and stimulates every tissue in the body by eliminating large quantities of carbon dioxide and making the blood rich with oxygen. The stomach, pancreas and liver are stimulated by the constant movements of the diaphragm, improving digestion.

The fast abdominal breathing in *kapalabhati* has a soothing and calming effect on the central nervous system and the autonomic nervous system. The blood circulation in the abdominal and the pelvic region is increased, which tones up the nerves and the muscles. It rejuvenates tired cells and nerves, keeping the face young, shining and wrinkle-free. *Kapalabhati* helps in awakening the *kundalini* power and induces alertness and inner awareness.

Caution: There should be no undue strain on the breathing mechanism at any stage of the practice of *vatakrama kapalabhati*. In the beginning, practise carefully under the expert guidance of a qualified teacher.

Do not practise if you have high blood pressure or lung disease. A hypertension or heart patient is advised not to resort to *kapalabhati* without expert supervision.

Do not retain the breath longer than is comfortable. Stop the practice if you feel dizzy.

Practice time: Daily. Beginners can start with three rounds of 15–20 rapid respirations.

Add ten respirations each week until you reach 120 respirations in each round, so that in the 12th week you are practising three rounds of 120 expirations.

Concentration: Navel centre (*manipura chakra*).

Method: Sit in a comfortable meditative posture. *Padmasana* is the best *asana* for practising *kapalabhati*, or *siddhasana* (for both these postures, see chapter 8). Press your palms moderately on your knees, and with your spine erect, close your eyes and relax.

Exhale and inhale quickly and lightly through both nostrils. Emphasize the exhalation (quick, strong and short). Your abdomen contracts, your diaphragm moves up into the thoracic area and pushes your lungs up. Allow the inhalation to come as a natural reflex (slow, lighter and longer). Your abdomen relaxes, your diaphragm descends down to the abdominal cavity, lowering the lungs with it.

In *kapalabhati* there is no resistance to breathing. Both the nostril and the glottis are wide open. The muscles of the neck and the face are kept relaxed so that the air escapes smoothly.

A greater number of respirations can be taken in *kapalabhati* than in *bhastrika pranayama* without hyperventilation occurring. Even ten minutes' practice of *kapalabhati* has been found to be physiologically harmless. Hyperventilation techniques of breathing are performed with the mouth. The breathing is fast and very deep at the frequency of 30–60 respirations per minute, causing an extreme wash-out of carbon dioxide and oversaturation of oxygen. *Kapalabhati*, on the other hand does not cause any abnormal situation like hyperventilation. The fast abdominal breathing in *kapalabhati* has a calming effect on the central and autonomic nervous system.

Tratak

Tratak means to gaze steadily with concentration at a fixed point without blinking. *Tratak* is a process of concentrating the mind and curbing its restless tendencies.

Benefits: The practice of *tratak* strengthens and cleanses the eyes, stimulates the nerve centres, is therapeutic in depression, insomnia, anxiety, poor concentration, and encourages strong, positive will-power and one-pointedness. Relieves eye ailments such as eyestrain, myopia, astigmatism and even early stages of cataract.

Practice time: *Tratak* can be practised at any time on a daily basis. Practise on an empty stomach. The most suitable time is between 4am and 6am after *asana* and *pranayama* practice. Or it can be practised late at night before meditation and retiring to bed.

Method: Practise in a darkened room. Sit in a comfortable meditation posture, with your head, neck and spine upright, but relaxed. Sit 3 feet away from a candle in front of you, with the flame at eye level. Make sure that the flame is not flickering from a draught.

Throughout the practice, keep your body still and your mind calm and quiet. Gaze at the mid-point of the flame for as long as possible without blinking and without strain until your eyes begin to water or become tired. In the beginning practise for about one minute and gradually increase to ten minutes. Then close the eyes and visualize the flame internally at the point between the eyebrows for one minute. If the after-image of the flame moves, bring it back to the centre and continue gazing until the image disappears.

As you concentrate on the candle flame do not allow your mind to wander. Observe your thoughts and feelings as they arise in your mind but do not become involved with them, just remain a silent witness to them.

When you have finished your practice, rub the palms of your hands together until you create heat in them. Place the warm palms over your eyes to relax and soothe them.

THE FOUR PURIFICATIONS

In addition to the classical *shatkarmas* are four purification techniques based on these which were devised by yogis to simplify and make safer the methods of purification.

These four purification techniques can be practised instead of the classical *shatkarmas* for purifying the *nadis* (subtle nerve channels), and for awakening the life energies in the body. The four purifications are:

1 *nadi shuddhi*
2 *kapalabhati*
3 *agni sara dhauti*
4 *ashwini mudra*

Practice time: The four purifications must be practised for two to three months before beginning the practice of *pranayama*, in the order given above.

Method: Throughout the practice, sit in a comfortable meditation posture keeping yourself upright and relaxed. With your eyes closed, concentrate on the mid-point between the eyebrows (the spiritual eye or *ajna chakra*).

1 **Nadi shuddhi:** Follow the method described on pages 190–2.
2 **Kapalabhati:** Follow the method described on pages 142–4.
3 **Agni sara dhauti:** Follow the method described on pages 119–20.
4 **Ashwini mudra:** Follow the method described on pages 159–60.

Fasting for Purification

Most people who practise yoga regularly find that it holds them to their correct weight, but basically the true yogi follows a diet that does not introduce too much waste matter into the body. Moderation is the keynote of a yogi's diet, and it means cutting down on all waste-producing drinks and foods that put a strain on the body's system, draining energy from the mind and body.

One of the first things to understand is that food is needed primarily to build up and maintain the body, but by about the age of 25 growth stops, ageing begins and only maintenance is needed. If the body is loaded with excess food or the wrong food, it will degenerate and age prematurely. Therefore food should be eaten in the right quantity and with the right quality to keep the body in a state of optimum health and balance. If you eat an excess of animal fats and proteins, ageing begins much faster. You can slow this ageing process down by practising the yoga techniques shown in this book on a regular basis: purification of the mind and body; the daily practice of yoga *asanas* and *pranayama*; meditating deeply every day; proper breathing; positive thinking; proper and sufficient rest and sleep; cultivating an optimistic and joyful outlook on life; regular exercise; and eating a vegetarian diet, with a moderate intake of food and fasting one day a week. These are all helpful vitalizing procedures that enliven the mind, body and soul.

To realize God, a sound body and a sound mind are essential. The body is a sacred temple and the mind controls the body. The soul, your true Self, which is conscious and luminous of itself, gives expression through the mind-body instrument. When the mind and body are purified of restricting mental and physical characteristics, the light of the soul can be self-revealed.

Fasting helps in keeping the body in an optimum state of health. Saints and monks of every order have used fasting with prayer and meditation to reach higher spiritual states of consciousness. Others have used it as a practice to improve their physical and mental health, while natural therapists recommend fasting as a basis of curing many diseases.

There is a difference between fasting and starving. Fasting is undertaken for religious or spiritual purposes, or to regain bodily health by detoxifying the body. It is giving up food when there is no real hunger, to eliminate toxins and poisons that the body's system has accumulated, and to allow nature to do its work of healing. In fact, the point where the body starts to starve because it has depleted its nutritional reserves is the end of the fast. From the beginning it is important to realize that the fasting stage only takes place so long as the body can support itself on the stored reserves within the body. Starvation begins when the body's reserves are depleted or at a dangerously low level.

BENEFITS OF FASTING

Fasting helps in removing toxins and poisons from the body, assisting in eliminating disease so that one can regain perfect health. Fasting is nature's own doctor.

By fasting, *prana* in the body is vivified and the life-spark rekindled.

Fasting purifies the *pranamaya kosha* (the vital sheath) and makes the mind serene and tranquil. It purifies the mind and takes one away from the body/ego-consciousness into the spiritual awareness and consciousness of the Self. The mood for prayer and meditation comes easily during a fast and the body feels lighter.

When there is no food being digested, the body can concentrate fully on what is already there. The build-up of waste materials is more effectively expelled via the bowels, kidneys, skin and lungs, purifying the blood. This in turn gives a wonderful feeling of lightness and freshness.

A complete fast for 24 hours gives the digestive system a chance to have a rest; the mind is free to contemplate the reality of God, meditate and pray.

Fasts of over one week not only cleanse the body but vivify one with more energy, power and spiritual strength. The will-power and concentration are developed, and all one's energies are thoroughly recouped. The body becomes firmed and the skin clearer, and the eyes sparkle like a baby's. The mind, insight and thoughts become clearer.

Spiritual Fasting

The Vedic scriptures point out that fasting helps one to control the mind and senses, so that one can advance in spiritual realization.

The most advanced yogis and saints fast inadvertently in that they actually forget to eat! This forgetfulness to eat is not the result of self-abnegation, but of spontaneous, pure love of God. Christ, Buddha and St Francis of Assisi, all fasted for 40 days before starting their divine missions.

In India, Ekadasi is observed on the 11th day after each full moon and the 11th day after each new moon. On these days yogis fast for God by concentrating their energies and attention towards spiritual activities like meditation, prayer, devotional chanting and observing silence.

There are different ways to observe Ekadasi. One may fast by drinking only pure water, or by eating only fruit. Devotees of Lord Krishna observe Ekadasi by abstaining from all grains and beans.

The *Brahma-Vaivarta Purana*, one of the oldest Vedic scriptures, states: 'One who observes Ekadasi is freed from all kinds of reactions to sinful activities and advances in pious life.'

The simple austerity of fasting on Ekadasi helps one to advance spiritually if it is carried out with faith and devotion. On the other hand, if one sacrifices eating simply for material reasons, one's sacrifices are denigrated by Lord Krishna, who says in the *Bhagavad Gita* (17:28), 'Sacrifices performed without faith in the Supreme are non-permanent. They are useless both in this life and the next.'

How to Fast

Do not fast if you have diabetes, are seriously toxic, with kidney disease, or have an eating disorder such as bulimia or anorexia (unless under medical, expert guidance). Also do not fast without expert guidance if you are recovering from serious alcohol or drug dependency.

The day before you fast eat lightly so that there is not much food to evacuate from the bowels. In the early morning of the day of the fast practise *laghoo shankhaprakshalana* (see page 130).

The duration of the fast depends largely on the purpose for which it is undertaken. For a general detoxification, one to three days a month is sufficient if you are following a balanced vegetarian diet. If you fast once a week the benefits will be greatly enhanced. Without guidance, the standard duration of three days is generally long enough to give the whole system a complete rest.

On a one- to three-day fast (a short fast) one can drink mineral water only or dilute pure fruit juice. On a pure fast one should take only pure mineral water, nothing else. It is good to drink plenty of water while fasting, as this increases the natural processes of purification. In a fast longer than two days, take pure mineral water with freshly pressed lemon juice (no added sugar, honey or sweetener) three times daily to aid in the cleansing process. Lemon juice is very good; it is a natural disinfectant for the stomach and a good cleanser for the liver and kidneys.

For a prolonged fast of up to one month I would suggest the grape fast, which is very purifying. There is an excellent book on grape fasting, *The Grape Cure* by Basil Shackleton, which is well worth reading. Fast on grapes, pure grape juice and pure mineral water only for two weeks, or for maximum benefit three or four weeks.

The grapes must be well washed in hot water to eliminate any chemicals that may have been sprayed on them. (Place grapes in a large bowl and wash with hot water three times, throwing the water away after each wash). Begin by eating a few ounces of grapes every few hours when you feel hungry. You must also eat the grape pips, as this will give you the needed roughage to keep the bowels working. Then you can gradually increase the amount from 2lb a day, up to 4 or 5lb a day.

On the first day of the fast your positive mental attitude will make all the difference to how you progress with it. Look upon fasting as a spiritual practice. Do not advertise it, let only those people know who are close to you, or who are sympathetic and understanding.

During the fast you will find that your tongue becomes thickly coated with a white or yellowish colour. This indicates that the process of cleansing is being accelerated to a great degree, and the toxins are being eliminated from the body. This coating will clear as you continue to fast. You can also help to clear the coating by cleaning the tongue with water and your fingers or toothbrush, as in *danta dhauti* (see page 136). Rinse your mouth out with water containing pure lemon juice and sea salt, then massage your gums and clean your teeth.

If you are having no bowel movement during the fast, then on each day of the fast choose one of the following options:

- Practise *laghoo shankhaprakshalana* (see page 130).
- Take powdered psyllium seeds. Mix a tablespoon of powder with half a pint of water in a blender, or whisk it by hand, and drink the mixture straight down. This gives a bulk which is not absorbed, but which clears the bowels, attracting toxic waste as it passes through the body.

Do not use laxatives!

While fasting try to rest by relaxing as much as possible. Do not practise any demanding, vigorous exercise or strenuous activities while fasting. Yoga postures, *pranayama*, taking walks in the fresh air, meditation and relaxation are all recommended during a fast.

Skin Brushing

The skin is an organ of elimination, as are the kidneys, liver and colon. Every day 1 lb of waste products is discharged through your skin. If the skin becomes inactive with its pores choked with dead cells, then uric acid and other impurities will remain in the body. Then the other eliminative organs, mainly the kidneys and the liver, will have to increase their work and will eventually become overworked. If toxins begin to build up in the tissues because the kidneys and liver cannot cope, then sooner or later disease will follow.

During a fast the eliminative organs, including the skin, are throwing off more toxins. To help this eliminative process and to keep a healthy and well-functioning skin we should take a few minutes every day to practise skin brushing.

To brush the skin take a moderately stiff, natural bristle brush. Keep it dry. Begin at the soles of your feet and work your way up your legs, your front and your back, brushing quite vigorously. After a week or so of daily brushing the skin will be less sensitive and more pressure can be used. But start off by using the brush very gently and gradually increase the pressure after the first few days. It is important that the bristles feel firm, as they help stimulate your blood circulation and lymphatic system. Then brush your hands and up your arm, followed by your chest (not the sensitive breasts) and upper back, with the brush strokes towards the heart. Do not brush your face, but go on to your neck and scalp.

Do not brush the sensitive parts of your body or skin affected by eczema.

Breaking the Fast

There is sometimes a tendency toward an abnormal craving to eat more food and all kinds of food after finishing a fast. Be very cautious and careful, for if you yield to these impulses, the consequences could be serious and harmful.

The method of breaking the fast will depend on its duration, but generally the first food taken should be liquid – diluted fruit juices and/or vegetable juice.

After a three-day fast drinking water only follow this procedure:

- On the fourth day, drink fruit and/or vegetable juice (dilute 50/50 with water).
- On the fifth day, eat fresh vegetable soup (no canned or packet soups!) and fresh fruit, but not at the same meal.

- On the sixth day, eat salad and a protein.
- On the seventh day, return to a normal vegetarian wholefood diet.

After a two, three or four-week fast, eating only grapes, the diet should then include two days of fruit and vegetable juices, live cultured yoghurt and grapes. Then continue the diet as for the fifth, sixth and seventh days of the three-day fast as above.

After breaking the fast it is also well to keep the following points in mind:

- Take only small amounts of food and chew each mouthful well. Eat with awareness.
- Your stomach will have shrunk and will require less food, so take care not to overload it.
- Do not over-exercise for the first few days.
- Drink plenty of pure mineral water.

The Yogic Diet

A vegetarian diet is essential for one who wants to follow a spiritual life. If you sincerely wish to progress and grow from the ordinary and materialistic life to a higher spiritual consciousness, then it becomes important to live on a vegetarian diet. For there are certain foods that help the mind and body to become more refined, and others that keep it down to the consciousness level of an animal.

The yogi selects and eats those foods which regenerate and impart vitality to the body with the minimum of waste and stress, and which leave the mind calm, clear and elevated.

Purification of the body and mind goes hand in hand with spiritual awakening. A vegetarian diet is highly conducive to sublime thoughts, divine contemplation, meditation and compassion.

The yogi has compassion and respect for all living things. This is reflected in the *Bhagavad Gita*:

> The humble sage, by virtue of knowledge, sees with equal vision, a learned brahmin [teacher-priest], a cow, an elephant, a dog and a dog-eater [outcast].

5:18

The yogi's diet is comprised of those foods which grow naturally – vegetables, herbs, fruits, nuts, seeds, grains, legumes (beans and pulses) and certain dairy products. The yogi consumes these foods either in their natural state or in a state that renders them fit for easy digestion with the minimum destruction of their *prana* (life-force).

OFFERING YOUR FOOD TO GOD

To be a vegetarian is good and is a step forward in purifying the mind and body, but to purify one's consciousness one needs to offer one's food to God with love and devotion, with the thought that God is tasting and blessing the food first. This will also help you to remember God every day: 'If one offers Me with love and devotion a leaf, a flower, fruit or water, I will accept it.' (*Bhagavad Gita* 9:26)

The preparation of food is also important. When one purchases, prepares and cooks food with awareness, care and love, *prana* is transmitted into the preparation. There is definitely a difference between the taste of food that has been cooked with love and that of food which has not.

Here is how you can prepare, cook and offer your food to God, bless it, and enjoy the eating of it.

First select natural, healthy vegetarian foods. Then wash your hands thoroughly as soon as you enter the kitchen. Wash the vegetables and fruit. In all preparations, use only fresh foods: do not mix leftovers in with the fresh food, for that which has been offered to the Lord should not be offered a second time. Try not to taste the food during preparation and cooking. We are cooking for God, offering our food to the Lord, so He should be first to taste it. Then when the food is nicely prepared with love and devotion, offer it back to the Source (God) from which everything emanates.

Now display the food attractively and sit quietly before it. If you are with your family or with spiritually minded friends, you can join hands and sit in meditation for one or two minutes with your eyes closed. Together you can repeat a prayer to God.

The one that I have used for many years is by my teacher, Sri Kriyananda (a direct disciple of Paramhansa Yogananda). You may like to use it, or perhaps make up your own.

> *Receive Lord in Thy light,*
> *The food we eat, for it is Thine,*
> *Infuse it with Thy love, Thy energy,*
> *Thy life divine.* Om, Amen.

After offering your food, enjoy eating it with awareness in silence. Eat slowly, chewing the food well before swallowing it. Remember, digestion begins in the mouth.

When you have finished your meal, sit for five or ten minutes in the *asana* called *vajrasana* (sitting on your heels with your hands relaxed on your knees). This posture diverts the blood supply from the legs to the stomach, aiding digestion.

BANDHAS

Bandha means 'lock', but it can also refer to a posture in which certain parts of the body are controlled or contracted in some way. It is very important to use *bandhas* in advanced *pranayama*, for without them you could injure the nervous system and possibly cause a pranic short-circuit in your body. To understand this, you need only a basic knowledge of an electrical circuit. Electricity is sent through a circuit which can work well and cause no harm so long as it has transformers, fuses, conductors and switches. Without these, the electric current going through it could be lethal. The *bandhas* 'lock' in the *prana* to prevent it being dissipated and direct the pranic energy or current to its destination, according to the concentration of the yogi. The *bandhas* also help to unite the *prana* and *apana* and direct this powerful pranic current into the *sushumna nadi*, to awaken the *kundalini shakti*. (*Apana* is *prana* [vital energy force] having a downward pranic air current. It operates in the region extending from below the navel to the anus. Its functions are to do with expulsion; it is responsible for the activity of ejaculation, defecation, urination, reproduction, digestion and childbirth delivery. *Apana* also carries the *kundalini* force upward in the *sushumna* to unite with *prana*.) What actually happens is that the *prana* is prevented from flowing upwards by *jalandhara bandha* (chin lock); and the *apana* is prevented from flowing downwards by *muladhara bandha* (anal lock). This causes the *prana* and *apana* to unite and flow into the *sushumna*.

JALANDHARA BANDHA (CHIN LOCK)

Jala means 'net' or 'network'. In the neck there is a network of nerves and arteries which go up to the brain. *Dhara* means 'pulling upwards'. When *jalandhara bandha* is applied, the internal and external carotid arteries, which lie on both sides of the neck and carry blood to the brain, are squeezed under pressure. *Jalandhara* also places pressure on the carotid sinus nerve. These pressures influence the blood pressure, slow down the heartbeat and slow down the nerve impulses to the brain. This brings calmness to the mind.

To practise *jalandhara bandha*, use the following procedure.

1 Sit in a comfortable posture, preferably *padmasana* or *siddhasana* (see chapter 8) (it is better to have the knees firmly on the floor) and place your palms on your knees. Close your eyes and relax.
2 Inhale deeply and retain the breath.
3 Without straining your neck muscles, bend your head forward and press your chin firmly into the hollow of your neck, between your collar bones. This gives a good stretch to the cervical vertebrae, which stimulates the nervous centres, frees the cranial nerves and beneficially affects the thyroid gland.
4 Hold this position for as long as comfortable without strain, then slowly release the chin lock by raising the head and exhale. Practise up to ten rounds, gradually increasing to 20. Do not inhale or exhale until the chin lock has been released and the head is upright.

Jalandhara bandha should not be practised by persons with high intra-cranial blood pressure or heart ailments without expert guidance.

From an esoteric point of view there is a subtle nectar that flows from the *sahasrara chakra* through the hole in the palate to the *manipura chakra* and is consumed by the gastric fire. *Jalandhara bandha* prevents this nectar from falling and so the elixir of life is stored and life itself is prolonged.

Jalandhara bandha can also be practised from a standing position, with the feet about 2 feet apart, the trunk leaning forward with the palms on the knees and the arms straight.

Uddiyana Bandha (Abdominal Lift)

Uddiyana comes from the Sanskrit root *ud* and *di*, which means 'flying up'. The pranic energy flies up through the *sushumna nadi* from the *manipura chakra* to the higher chakras.

It can be practised either standing or sitting. For beginners it is best to start practising from a standing position, because it is easier to accomplish in this position.

1. Stand with your feet about 2 feet apart.
2. With your knees slightly bent, grip the middle of your thighs with your hands and lean your trunk forward from the waist.
3. Look forward as you inhale deeply, then exhale completely. Slowly drop your head forward and rest your chin in the hollow of your throat.
4. Contract and pull your whole abdominal region back towards your spine, lifting it upwards. Raise your lumbar and dorsal spine forward and upwards.
5. Retain your breath out holding the *bandha* for as long as is comfortable. On no account strain or go beyond your endurance.
6. To release the *bandha* relax the abdominal muscles first. Then slowly raise your head and inhale slowly.
7. Return to normal relaxed breathing for a few breaths, then repeat the whole process again. In the beginning practise three to five abdominal lifts, gradually increasing to ten in each held breath.

Practise on an empty stomach. Early morning on rising is the best time.

Release the chin lock before inhalation. Do not practise if you have high blood pressure, hiatus hernia (hernia of the diaphragm), ulcers or heart ailments. Women should not practise during pregnancy or menstruation.

The benefits of *uddiyana bandha* are:

- It increases the gastric fire.
- The abdominal organs and glands are toned.
- The adrenal glands are normalized.
- When combined with *nauli kriya* it acts as a gastro-intestinal tonic and eliminates constipation.

- It alleviates indigestion and abdominal diseases.
- It stimulates the sympathetic nerves of the solar plexus and *manipura chakra*.
- It bestows youth and vitality.
- It exercises the diaphragm vigorously.
- It massages the heart without strain.

MULABANDHA (ANAL LOCK)

The Sanskrit word *mula* means 'root' and refers to the region between the anus and the genitals (the perineum). *Mulabandha* is practised in conjunction with *pranayama* and *mudras*.

1 Sit in a comfortable meditation posture, preferably *siddhasana* or *siddha yoni asana* (see chapter 8), because these *asanas* improve the effect of the *bandha* by the heel being pressed against the perineum.
2 Inhale slowly and deeply.
3 Retain the breath with *jalandhara bandha*.
4 Simultaneously contract the internal and external anal sphincter muscles. This may seem difficult at first, but if you first bring your awareness to the anus and contract it, then concentrate on a point just above this sphincter muscle (perineum) and contract it, you will find that it is not so difficult. Simultaneously draw the *apana* upward by contracting the abdominal muscles.
5 The breath is retained internally holding both *mulabandha* and *jalandhara bandha* in order to unite the *prana* and *apana*.
6 Release the contraction of both the internal and external sphincter muscles. Then slowly release the *jalandhara bandha*, by raising the head and exhale.

Mulabandha can also be held with external breath retention. The breath retention, internal or external, is held for as long as comfortable. Do not strain. It would be helpful for beginners to practice *ashwini mudra* first before attempting *mulabandha* (see pages 159–60).

The benefits of this practice are:

- It increases the benefit of *pranayama* during retention (*kumbhak*).

- It strengthens the reproductive glands.
- It generates vitality and helps in awakening *kundalini*.
- It strengthens the sphincter muscles of the anus.
- It enables one to maintain celibacy.
- It stimulates the gastric fire.
- It relieves constipation and piles.

MAHABANDA (TRIPLE LOCK)

In *mahabandha*, the three bandhas – *mulabandha*, *uddiyana bandha* and *jalandhara bandha* – are practised simultaneously during external retention of the breath in *pranayama*.

1 Sit in *siddhasana* or *siddha yoni asana* with your palms on your knees.
2 Inhale deeply and exhale deeply.
3 Perform *mulabandha, uddiyana bandha*, then *jalandhara bandha* in that order.
4 Retain your breath, holding the three *bandhas* for as long as is comfortable. Do not strain.
5 Release the *bandhas* in reverse order: *jalandhara, uddiyana* then *mulabandha*.
6 Inhale slowly and relax.

Mahabandha vitalizes the whole body with *prana*, stimulates the psychic energy flow and combines all the benefits of the three individual *bandhas*.

MUDRAS

The Sanskrit word *mudra* means 'to seal'. The *Gheranda Samhita* describes 25 *mudras* and *bandhas*, many of which can only be practised under the expert guidance of a guru. Among these are 12 that are important, some of which I have already covered under '*Bandhas*' above.

Mudras give both mental and physical benefits, but are primarily used to invoke a spiritual mood. They prepare the mind for meditation and serve to control and direct the pranic forces within the body.

PASHINEE MUDRA (THE FOLDED MUDRA)

1. Lie down on your back, raise your legs together to touch the floor behind your head. This is the plough posture (*halasana*).
2. Now separate your feet about hip-width apart. Bend your legs at the knees and bring your thighs in towards the chest, until your knees touch your ears, shoulders and the floor.
3. Clasp your arms tightly around the back of your knees. Breathe deeply and slowly with your concentration on the breath in the navel centre.
4. Hold the posture for as long as comfortable, then release the pose and relax.

Be careful not to strain the back muscles. Do not practise if you suffer from sciatica, high blood pressure or detached retina. Females should not practice during menstruation.

The benefits of this posture are that it balances the nervous system, stretches the back muscles and stimulates the spinal nerves. It also massages the abdominal organs and tones the sexual organs.

ASHWINI MUDRA (HORSE MUDRA)

This *mudra* is so called because, after a horse has evacuated its stools, it then dilates and contracts the anus several times.

Stage 1

1. First lie down on your back and bend your knees, with your feet about hip-width apart and flat on the floor. Keep your back flat on the floor. In this position the abdomen is relaxed, which makes it easier for the next stage.
2. Now contract and release the anal sphincters, which are situated at the rectum.

Practise this contraction and releasing a number of times, then relax.

Stage 2

1. Now sit up into a comfortable meditative posture, close your eyes and relax.
2. Inhale deeply and retain your breath.
3. Contract your anal sphincter for a few seconds.
4. Exhale and release the contraction.
5. Relax for a few seconds then repeat the whole process a few more times.

Stage 3

1. Still sitting in a meditative posture, inhale deeply and retain the breath.
2. Contract and release the anal sphincter rapidly and repeatedly for as many times as you can hold your breath comfortably.
3. Relax the contraction and exhale.

Start with three rounds of 30 contractions each, gradually increasing this number to ten rounds of 60 each. Be careful not to strain.

The benefits of *ashwini mudra* are:

- It strengthens the pelvic floor, preventing prolapse of the rectum and uterus.
- It prevents haemorrhoids (piles) by toning the veins of the anus.
- It prevents constipation by stimulating intestinal peristalsis.
- It tones up the seminal glands and nerves in the pelvic area.
- It strengthens *mulabandha* and forces the *prana* upward.

Note that *mulabandha* differs from *ashwini mudra* in that there is no alternate contraction and dilation of the sphincter.

MAHA MUDRA (THE GREAT SEAL)

This is the most important *mudra*. It forces the *prana* upward and aids in awakening the *kundalini*.

1. Sit on the floor with both your legs outstretched.

2 Fold your left leg and press the left heel against your anus. Extend your right leg forward and grasp your toe with both hands. Keep the leg straight.
3 Inhale deeply and retain the breath, applying both *mulabandha* and *jalandhara bandha*.
4 Retain the breath for as long is comfortable while keeping your inward gaze at the point between the eyebrows (*ajna chakra*).
5 Release *jalandhara*, then *mulabandha* and exhale very slowly.
6 Repeat the whole process with your right heel pressed against your anus.
7 In the beginning practise two mudras on each side, gradually increasing to ten.

Another variation is to stretch your trunk forward while holding the toes.

If you cannot fold your leg right under your buttocks so that you are pressing the heel against your anus, then you can practise *siddhasana* or *siddha yoni asana* with the heel pressed against the perineum.

The benefits of this practice are:

1 It stimulates the flow of pranic energy.
2 It prevents haemorrhoids (piles), constipation, enlargement of the spleen and abdominal disorders.
3 It calms the mind and body, preparing one for meditation.

MAHA VEDHA MUDRA (GREAT PIERCING *MUDRA*)

In this *mudra* the chakras and *nadis* are pierced by the consciousness.

1 Sit in *padmasana* (see chapter 8) with your palms resting flat on the floor beside your buttocks.
2 Inhale deeply and slowly.
3 Retain the breath and apply *mulabandha* and *jalandhara bandha*. Concentrate on *ajna chakra*.
4 Raise your body from the floor by balancing on your hands and gently drop your buttocks against the floor.
5 Release the *bandhas* and exhale slowly.

Start with two rounds, gradually increasing to ten.

A variation for those that cannot sit in *padmasana* is to sit with the left heel pressed against the anus, and the right foot on the left thigh. In the same way you can place the palms by your sides on the floor and raise the buttocks slowly, then drop them against the floor.

In terms of benefit there is not much difference between *maha mudra*, *maha vedha mudra* and *mahabandha*.

Yoga Mudra (Yogic seal)

1 Sit in *padmasana* (lotus pose – see chapter 8). If you are unable to do this, then sit in half-lotus, *siddhasana* or even *vajrasana*. Close your eyes and relax.
2 Bring your hands behind your back and hold your right wrist with your left hand.
3 Inhale slowly and deeply, feeling the consciousness rise with the breath from the *muladhara chakra* to the *ajna chakra*.
4 Retain your breath for a few seconds with your concentration at the *ajna chakra*.
5 Slowly bend your head and trunk forwards as you slowly exhale, extending the whole of the front of your trunk.
6 Rest your forehead on the floor and relax into the pose, breathing normally, with your concentration on the *ajna chakra*.
7 Hold the pose for as long as is comfortable. Be careful not to strain your knees, ankles or back muscles.
8 Inhale as you come back up.

Start by holding this pose for one or two minutes, and gradually increase the duration to 15 minutes or more.

The benefits of *yoga mudra* are:

1 It increases the memory.
2 It stimulates the gastric fire.
3 It massages the abdominal organs.
4 It stretches the spine and tones the spinal nerves.
5 It tones the lungs and heart.
6 It awakens the *manipura chakra* (navel centre).

7 It prevents constipation and indigestion by increasing assimilation and elimination.

VAJROLI MUDRA (THUNDERBOLT *MUDRA*)

This is a very advanced *mudra*; in fact it is an important *yoga kriya* and requires a very high stage of control over the sexual organs. *Vajroli* consists of several stages, in one of which a silver tube (catheter) is inserted 12 inches into the urethra. Then water is sucked up through this tube, and when this is perfected milk, oil and honey can be sucked up. At the final stage the urethral control is attained and the yogi is able to suck up fluids into the bladder via the urethra without the silver tube. Even air can be sucked inside via the urethra.

These stages are practised under the expert and experienced guidance of a guru. It is a very advanced practice and in the beginning the silver catheter is only inserted 1 inch into the urethra and gradually increased to 2 inches and so on up to 12 over a period of time. The object of *vajroli mudra* is to gain perfect control over the sexual organs and to preserve the semen. To practise this advanced technique one would have to observe strict celibacy.

There is, however, a simple technique which can be used.

1 Sit in a comfortable meditative *asana*, placing your hands on your knees and closing your eyes.
2 Draw your sexual organs upwards by tensing and pulling the lower abdomen and contracting the sexual organs – the testes in the male and the vagina in the female. Do not strain or over-exert the contraction.
3 While contracting the sexual organs concentrate on the *swadisthana chakra*.
4 Release the contraction and relax.

VIPARITA KARANI MUDRA (REVERSE POSTURE *MUDRA*)

1 Lie on your back with the arms at your sides.
2 Inhale slowly and raise your trunk to a 45-degree angle with your legs at 90 degrees. Support your body by cupping your hips in the

palms of your hands, with your elbows rested on the floor. Your whole body should be relaxed, with your eyes closed.
3. Apply *kechari mudra* (see pages 164–6) and inhale throughout this practice with *ujjayi pranayama* (see chapter 5).
4. Inhale slowly from the *manipura chakra* to the *vishuddhi chakra*.
5. Exhale, maintaining awareness at the *vishuddhi chakra*.
6. Inhale again from the *manipura chakra* to the *vishuddhi chakra*.
7. Continue breathing in this way for as long as is comfortable, then exhale and come down to relax.

Of all the inverted poses, *viparita karani* is the easiest to perform. You may experience some discomfort to the elbows, which can be lessened by practising on a folded blanket. It is said that the sun dwells at the root of the navel and the moon at the root of the palate. In *viparita karani mudra* this process is reversed, bringing the sun upward and the moon downward.

In the beginning practise this *mudra* for only a minute, then gradually increase to five minutes or more. It is said in the yogic treatises that if a yogi practises this *mudra* for three hours daily, he conquers death. It is also said that if one practises for three hours daily for six months wrinkles on the face and grey hair disappear.

This practice has the following benefits:

- It removes congestion of the spleen and liver.
- It prevents constipation, haemorrhoids, prolapse of the organs in the abdomen and dyspepsia.
- It increases vitality.
- It preserves the subtle nectar that flows from the *sahasrara chakra*, and so rejuvenates and purifies the body.
- It sublimates sexual energy from the lower chakras to the higher.
- It corrects the adverse effects of improper *pranayama*.
- It diverts the flow of blood to the thyroid glands, promoting their health and increasing their vitality.

However, it should not be practised until at least three hours after a meal; and you should wait half an hour after strenuous exercise, or until the body is rested, before attempting it. It should also not be practised by women during the menstrual period, nor by people with high blood pressure, enlarged thyroid or serious heart problems.

KECHARI MUDRA (TONGUE LOCK)

The Sanskrit *kha* means *akasha* ('space'), and *chari* means 'to remove'. So *kechari mudra* means 'moving-in-space position'. Through practising *kechari mudra* the consciousness dwells in *akasha*, the space between the astral and the physical.

The *Hatha Yoga Pradipika* refers to *kechari* as 'the greatest of all *mudras*' and says that one who perfects *kechari* can overcome sleep, hunger, thirst, disease, old age and death.

The traditional practice of *kechari* by very advanced yogis in India, under the direction and guidance of a guru, involves having the lower membrane of the tongue (fraenum linguae) gradually cut over a period of months, until the membrane that connects the tongue with the lower part of the mouth is severed. The reason for this is to make the tongue as long as necessary, so that when it is retroverted it can be made to enter the upper back cavity, above the palate. The tip of the tongue is pressed towards the eyebrow centre, where the three *nadis*, *sushumna*, *ida* and *pingala*, join.

Some very advanced yogis with the retroverted tongue in *kechari mudra* actually close the rima glottidis (a narrow triangular fissure or cleft between the inferior or true vocal cords in front and the bases and vocal processes of the arytenoid cartilages behind). This completely closes the air passage and controls the impulse to breathe in, so that the period of breath suspension can be lengthened.

Advanced yogis of this technique with perfect control over their mind and body have been known to sit perfectly still and suspend the breath for 40 days.

In his *14 Steps to Joy*, Sri Kriyananda says:

> The positive and negative energies in the tongue and nasal passages, when joined together, create a cycle of energy in the head, which instead of allowing the energy to flow outward to the body, generates a magnetic field that draws energy upward from the body and from the base of the spine to the brain.

CAUTION: Under *no* circumstances cut the membrane of the tongue. It is definitely *not* recommended. Sri Kriyananda related a true story of how his guru, Paramhansa Yogananda spoke severely against this practice at one time, when one of his students began to cut the membrane of the tongue to lengthen it.

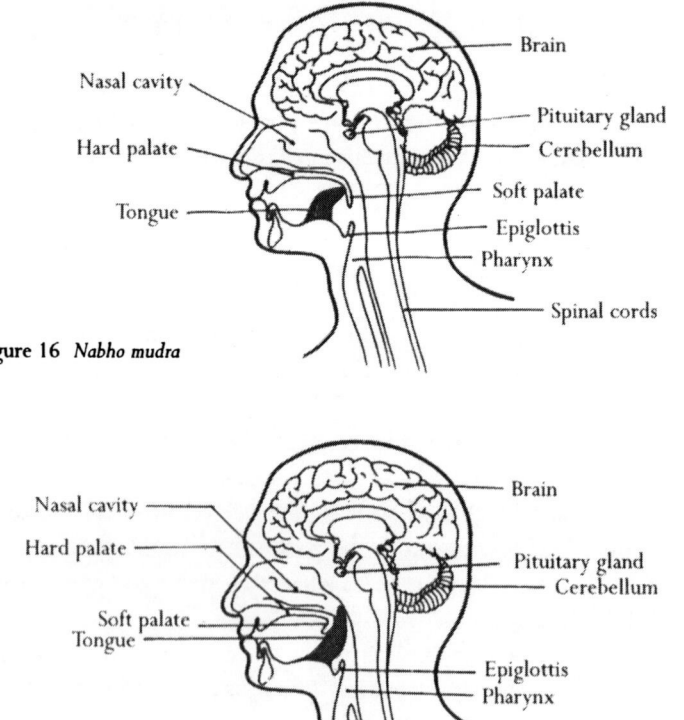

Figure 16 *Nabho mudra*

Figure 17 *Kechari mudra*

Within the tongue there are five main nerves, blood vessels and arteries, mucous glands and lymphatic vessels. To cut the fraenum of the tongue could sever nerves, making the tongue go numb and could also leave it without a proper blood supply.

The practice described here is a safer version of *kechari*, *without* cutting the tongue.

Exercises to Stretch the Tongue

1. First, turn your tongue back and touch your uvula (the fleshy grape-like structure that hangs down from the back of your soft palate). Look in a mirror as you practise, to see what is happening.

2 Turn your tongue backwards and reach the uvula with the underside. With your mouth closed, push the base of your tongue up towards the roof of your mouth until you feel a stretch underneath your fraenum. Gently but firmly practise without straining. Practise as often as you want to.
3 Place the top side of your tongue up against the roof of your mouth, and press it there. Then create a suction by sucking your tongue hard to the roof of the mouth.

  Now, gently open your mouth, still with your tongue sucked up against the roof of the mouth, until you feel the fraenum being stretched.

  The final position of this exercise involves opening the mouth wider, so that the suction is released, and the tongue falls forward making a 'plucking' sound.

  Practise this 50 to 100 times daily.
4 Take a fine, clean, damp cloth. Stick your tongue out, grasp it with the cloth and 'milk' it by pulling on it gently and massaging it, to stretch it. This is called *dohana*.

  Practise this for two or three minutes daily.
5 With your fingers, gently but firmly push the tip of the tongue backwards until you feel the fraenum being stretched. This is called *chalana*.
6 Grasp your tongue and gently brush your fraenum against the bottom teeth.

  Practise this for one to two minutes daily.

Nabho Mudra (Sky Mudra)

This is a simple version of *kechari mudra*.
1 Sit in a comfortable meditative posture, relax your body and close your eyes.
2 With your mouth closed, roll your tongue back, so that the lower surface touches your upper palate. Without straining, draw the tip of your tongue as far back as possible, and press it upward against the back part of the mouth.

  Retain this position while practising *ujjayi pranayama* (see chapter 5). Practise for as long as comfortable, then relax the tongue.

Kechari Mudra: **The Full Practice**

In this practice, the tongue goes behind the uvula (the soft palate) and is inserted into the nasal cavity. The tip of the tongue presses upward and forward, stimulating certain nerves in that area. Breathing is performed through the nose, because the mouth is blocked by the tongue.

The tongue in this position actually creates a short-circuit from energy in the medulla oblongata (base of brain) and directs it to the eyebrow centre (spiritual eye). Normally, the energy enters through the medulla oblongata, then comes down and goes out through the body.

This helps to awaken the *kundalini* and higher states of consciousness. It purifies the body and brings calmness to the mind.

With daily practice of the tongue-stretching exercises it can take three to six months for the tongue to lengthen.

YONI MUDRA

Yoni mudra induces a state of *pratyahara* (sense withdrawal).

1. Sit in a comfortable meditative posture, preferably *siddhasana*. Relax your body and close your eyes.
2. Inhale deeply and slowly, then retain the breath.
3. Close your ears with your thumbs, pressing lightly over the tragus of each ear (the tragus is the fleshy prominence in front of the opening). Close your eyes, with your index fingers lightly pressing over the outer corners of the closed eyelids. Close your nostrils with your middle fingers and place your third fingers above, and your little fingers below your lips to close the mouth.
4. While holding your breath with *yoni mudra*, inwardly gaze at the point between your eyebrows (*ajna chakra*). Concentrate on this point and try to see the spiritual eye of the opalescent blue, surrounded by a gold circle of light. In the centre of the blue is a tiny five-pointed silvery-white shining star. Dive deep into this star and meditate. Listen for any inward sounds, as this is also a technique of Nada Yoga.
5. Retain your breath for as long as is comfortable, then release your fingers and exhale.

5

PRANAYAMA

Pranayama is a Sanskrit word formed by two words. *Prana* means a subtle life-force which gives energy to the mind and body, and *ayama* signifies the voluntary effort to control and direct this *prana*.

Pranayama is essentially a process by which *prana* is controlled by regulating the breathing voluntarily. It involves a temporary pause or interval in the movement of breath.

The basic movements of *pranayama* are *rechak* (exhalation), *purak* (inhalation), and *kumbhak* (retention of the breath).

Having instructed us in the mastery of the meditation posture (*asana*), by being steadily and firmly seated with the mind or attention flowing in one direction, Patanjali now proceeds with *pranayama*, which he deals with in five sutras (49–53, *Sadhana Pada*).

> *Having established a firm, steady posture, one then regulates the life-force* (prana) *by natural voluntary suspension of the breath after inhalation and exhalation – this is* pranayama.
>
> *Yoga Sutras* 2:49

In this sutra he is saying, 'Exhale and retain the breath.' This does not mean exhale, inhale and hold the breath, but rather that if you breathe out and then refuse to inhale again, you will very soon experience what *prana* is. It jumps quickly into activity when you are forced to inhale another breath. What makes you take the next breath after holding it out for so long is *prana*.

Please try it, for no definition can ever show you *prana* as clearly as one moment's experience. If you want to know what total absorption of the mind is, exhale and suspend the breathing. You will find that during that period, you will think of nothing except your breath. It is not possible to think of anything else at all. A few seconds will seem like half an hour.

The Hatha yogis' explanation of this is that it is the breath (or the movement of *prana*) that enables your mind to think. If this is suspended, then the mind loses its fuel, and so it is no longer distracted, it becomes quiet.

During deep meditation the breath naturally becomes suspended for a short period of time, and it is this interval that constitutes *pranayama*. To the meditator in such deep meditation, there is no sense of time; the mind is still, and in that deep peace, there is joy or bliss.

> The variations in pranayama are external, internal or suspended. The interval is regulated by place, duration and number, and becomes progressively prolonged and subtle.
>
> Yoga Sutras 2:50

In this sutra Patanjali describes three types of *pranayama* on the basis of the nature of the interval that causes a temporary suspension of breath.

- a pause after a very slow and prolonged exhalation (*bahya kumbhaka* – external breath retention)
- a pause after a deep, prolonged inhalation (*abhyantara kumbhaka* – internal breath retention)
- a prolonged pause in between the inhalation and exhalation

In this technique, he says the interval is regulated by place, duration and number.

- *Place* refers to where the breath is held (external, internal or suspended).
- *Duration* refers to the duration of the breath retention.
- *Number* means the ratio between inhalation, retention and exhalation of the breath.

> The fourth type of pranayama is the spontaneous suspension of the breath, that occurs while concentrating on something external or internal.
>
> Yoga Sutras 2:51

This spontaneous suspension of the breath (known as *keval kumbhaka*) is

experienced by the practitioner at any time without any effort. It comes automatically after prolonged practice of *pranayama*.

> The attainment of pranayama removes mental darkness and ignorance, which veils the inner light of the soul ... And the mind attains the power to concentrate.
>
> Yoga Sutras 2:52–3

The benefits of *pranayama* are given in these two sutras. If you practise *pranayama* efficiently and effectively, the veil of dark ignorance that covers the inner light is removed. *Pranayama* aids contemplation and removes distraction from the mind, so that it becomes easy to concentrate and meditate.

Throughout the *Yoga Sutras*, there is a simple but very important message for us to remember: 'Practise yoga in order that these obstacles [of the mind] may be removed.' When the obstacles are removed, then the Self (Seer) rests in its own true nature and life becomes enlightened.

PRANA, THE VITAL ENERGY OF THE UNIVERSE

> When there is prana in the body, it is called life; when it leaves the body, it results in death. So one should practise pranayama.
>
> Yogi Svatmarama, Hatha Yoga Pradipika 2:3

The Sanskrit word *prana* translates as 'first unit of life-force'. There are many terms used for it, including 'vital energy', 'breath of life' and 'life-force'. Paramhansa Yogananda translated it as 'lifetrons', in essence, condensed thoughts of God or substance of the astral world.

Paramhansa Yogananda developed a God-inspired system of 39 'energization exercises' to recharge the brain and body with cosmic energy (*prana*) directly. Those devotees who follow his path of Kriya Yoga and practise these recharging exercises know the secret of recharging and energizing the body at will, at any time or place, with *prana*, the electric life-current given to us by God.

Prana is the link between the astral and physical bodies. When this link is broken or cut off, then the astral body separates from the physical body, and what we call death takes place. The *prana* departs from the physical body and is withdrawn into the astral body. Similarly, if a car battery is disconnected from a motor car engine, or any electrical appliance is disconnected from the electric power supply, the motor car or the electrical appliance are of no use, they are dead without the electric current flowing through them.

Everything in the human, animal and plant kingdoms, is dependent on the air it breathes to live. Life, *prana* and breath are intimately connected. There is not one life form that can survive, or even move, without the current of energy called *prana*.

> When the breath [prana] is restless, the mind also becomes unsteady, but when the breath is still, so is the activity of the mind. Then a yogi attains a complete motionless state of consciousness (chitta). One should therefore restrain one's breath.
>
> Yogi Svatmarama, *Hatha Yoga Pradipika* 2:2

Prana is intimately related to the mind and mental processes; one cannot move without the other also moving. When there is turbulence in the mind, the breath becomes restless and vice versa — the breath (movement of *prana*) also affects the mind and its mental processes.

We need only to be aware of emotions such as anger, fear, hatred and jealousy to feel what effect it has on our breathing. When we become angry or emotionally upset, our breathing is markedly changed in its rate and depth. For example, when we become angry, the breath becomes faster and we lose control over it and over our mind. Anger agitates and shatters the whole nervous system, and can also lead to hatred, which is even worse; for when the heart is attuned to hate it is impossible to feel attunement with God, who is love.

The emotions and the mental processes are related to the nervous system and through it they change our breathing. That is why it is important to develop positive attitudes and positive thoughts, and to change or overcome unwanted negative or destructive tendencies and behaviours. How? By developing the virtues we associate with divine qualities: love, inner joy, compassion, selflessness, kindness, generosity, loyalty, gentleness, forgiveness, peacefulness, calmness and contentment.

When these virtues are naturally and spontaneously expressed, then the energy naturally and continuously flows in abundance. The *prana* in an upward flow permeates the whole body, elevating the consciousness. Conversely, if we become negative in our thoughts, attitudes and behaviour or suppress our natural feelings, the pranic flow of energy sinks downward, the energy becomes concentrated in the lower part of the body. The body and mind become depressed and the breath unstable.

The practice of *pranayama* helps in transforming the total personality by clearing mental obstructions, purifying the subtle channels (*nadis*) through which *pranas* flow, awakening dormant vital forces in the body, focusing the attention, developing concentration and improving overall health and vitality.

> *By the proper and careful practice of* pranayama *one attains optimum health, a peaceful, steady mind and a firm and lustrous body free from disease.*
> Yogi Svatmarama, *Hatha Yoga Pradipika* 2:16–18

Pranayama aims primarily at controlling the mind and suspending the mental activity and ego-consciousness (the seat of *vrittis* – *see* below) in order to bring about a still mind. With the mind still and the breathing calm, the inner light of the true Self shines radiantly. The light of the Self is always pure, even though it is tinted by the coloured filters of the mind. When the coloured filters are removed, there is only one pure light, the true Self.

Vrittis – Instincts, Urges and Desires

Vrittis translates as 'fluctuations', 'modifications of the mind', 'waves', 'thought waves', 'mental whirlpool'.

The mind which exists in the astral body is called *antahkarana* (inner instrument). It contains four main elements:

- *manas* (mind) – thinking, willing, doubting, recording faculty of the mind
- *buddhi* (intellect) – discriminating and decision-making faculty of the mind, and intuitive wisdom
- *ahamkara* (ego) – self-arrogating part of the mind which sees itself as separate from God and others; identifying faculty of the mind
- *chitta* (subconscious) – the storehouse of past experiences; memory; 'mind-stuff', mind-field

The *chitta* or 'mind-stuff' is a composite of three primordial energies in creation. These three energies or attributes of nature (*prakriti*), are called *gunas* (qualities):

- *sattva* – quality of truth, purity, light
- *rajas* – quality of passion, energy, desire
- *tamas* – quality of ignorance, inertia, darkness

Like three intertwined cords in a rope the *gunas* pulsate in the mind, one more vibrant or dormant than the other at a given time. They interact in various degrees on each other giving us the experience of happiness and fulfilment, pleasure and pain, and lack of energy and indifference.

When the mind is of a sattvic nature it performs good actions, it is virtuous, peaceful, calm, joyful and selfless.

When the mind is of a rajasic nature it is egotistical, absorbed in worldly and selfish interests. It is restless with desires.

When the mind is of a tamasic nature it is careless, ignorant, lethargic, negative, depressive, dull and selfish.

The *chitta* is very much like a lake on which waves rise and fall. These waves are the innumerable thoughts that give existence to the mind. Without these 'thought waves' (*vrittis*) the mind cannot survive, it has no existence. The mind clings to that with which it identifies, thinking that its security comes from there. It thinks, feels and directs the senses to act accordingly. The 'I' (*ahamkara*) gives the motive power to the instincts in the mind, which generates desires in relationship to objects through an outward projection, and registers them inwardly as memory, by experience for later reference.

The innumerable *vrittis* that are rising and falling in each moment within the mind-field (*chitta*) can be divided into five main categories, called *kleshas* (afflictions).

Kleshas are of two kinds:

- *klishta* (afflicted, painful, distressing)
- *aklishta* (not afflicted; non-painful, pleasing)

These are the five main causes of suffering in life as given by Patanjali in his *Yoga Sutras*, 2:3–9.

1 ignorance (*avidya*)
2 I-am-ness (*asmita*)
3 attraction (*raga*)
4 aversion (*dvesha*)
5 fear of death/clinging to life (*abhinivesha*)

First there is ignorance (*avidya*), the source of all the other obstacles. The meaning of ignorance here is to ignore the truth of our spiritual identity – a lack of inner awareness of the eternal, blissful, conscious, divine Self. Ignorance creates delusion, which covers the knowledge of the Self. Without experiencing our own true eternal nature, we cannot realize that this same divine Self exists in all creatures. In ignorance we create a sense of separateness from each other and from God.

I-am-ness or ego (*asmita*) is identification of the self with the body, mind and senses. It is forgetfulness of our true divine nature.

In this forgetfulness we experience ourselves as finite, limited and temporal.

Attraction (*raga*) is the restless pursuit of pleasure; attraction to the objects of the senses. It is also confusion of wants and needs.

Aversion (*dvesha*) is a dislike or avoidance of that which brings unhappiness and suffering.

Patanjali's fifth *klesha*, fear of death (*abhinivesha*), is the tenacious clinging to life, not wanting to let go of the ego. It is resistance to change.

Clinging to life is the habit of dependence on objective sources for enjoyment and happiness, and fear of losing them. The greatest fear is death, fearing that we will cease to exist and lose our identity.

Patanjali gives us the remedy for overcoming these five afflictions (*kleshas*). (*Yoga Sutras* 2:10–11). He informs us that these afflictions may be subtle or gross. To reduce or eliminate the subtle afflictions one has to reverse the energy of the thought responsible for each affliction, back to its source or cause in the ego, and purify it with its own true opposite. For example, if the feeling of attraction or repulsion enters the mind, then substitute it with contentment or acceptance.

The gross, active and outward expressions of the five afflictions can be silenced through meditation.

Another remedy Patanjali gives to us, (*Yoga Sutras* 2:26) is the unwavering practice of uninterrupted awareness, discriminating between what is real and what is unreal. This is the means to remove ignorance.

Patanjali then tells us (*Yoga Sutras* 2:27–28) that the impurities of the mind are diminished and that we can attain the highest stage of enlightenment through the dedicated practice of the seven limbs of yoga (*samadhi*, being the eighth limb).

Self-realization is attained by discrimination, dispassion, determination, unbroken awareness, whole-hearted dedication to the practice of yoga and meditation. The mind has to be purified and made one-pointed. It takes patience, perseverance, and a burning aspiration for truth to succeed on the spiritual path.

THE FIVE LIFE-FORCES OF THE BODY

The movements of *prana* are not only those which enter this body through the vehicle of the breath. There are movements of *prana* also within one's own body. These *pranas* are called *vayus* (vital airs); they are the intelligent life-forces which are manifested in the astral body and function through the five subsidiary nerve centres in the brain and spinal cord.

THE FIVE MAJOR *VAYUS*

- *Udana vayu* functions in the body above the larynx (throat) and the top of the head. It controls the automatic functions of the cephalic divisions of the autonomic nervous system. It controls speech, the sense of balance, memory and intellect. *Udana* has an upward movement – it carries *kundalini* to the *sahasrara*, and separates the astral body from the physical body at the time of death. *Udana* is a pale white colour.
- *Prana vayu* functions in the region between the larynx and the base of the heart. It uses the autonomic nervous system controlling speech, the respiratory muscles, blood circulation and body temperature. *Prana* is the colour of blood, or a rose pink like that of a coral.
- *Samana vayu* functions between the heart and the navel region, maintaining a balance between *apana* and *vayu*. Through the

sympathetic part of the autonomic system, it controls all the metabolic activity involved in digestion. *Samana* is a colour somewhere between that of milk and crystal, which shines.
- *Apana vayu* functions in the region from the navel to the feet. It has a downward movement normally, but carries the *kundalini shakti* upwards in *sushumna* to unite with *prana*. *Apana* controls the functions of the kidneys, excretory system, colon, rectum and sex organs through the autonomic system. *Apana* is a colour between white and red.
- *Vyana vayu* permeates throughout the whole body and is the aura around the body. It helps the other *vayus* to function properly. It controls both the voluntary and involuntary movements of the muscles and joints. It keeps the whole body upright by generating unconscious reflexes along the spine. In addition to this, it controls the physical nerves and the subtle astral nerves (*nadis*). *Vyana* is the colour of a ray of light.

The Five Minor *Pranas*

- *Naga* controls the function of belching and hiccoughing. It also gives rise to consciousness.
- *Kurma* controls the function of opening the eyelids and causes vision.
- *Karikara* controls sneezing and induces hunger and thirst.
- *Devadatha* controls yawning.
- *Dhananjaya* causes the decomposition of the body after death.

Guidelines for the Practice of *Pranayama*

Place

Select a clean, warm, airy place to practise in, a room where you can sit quietly without being disturbed. If you can sit outside, then make sure that you are warm, away from pollution, noise and distractions.

Time

Pranayama is best commenced in spring (especially after doing a 'spring cleansing' such as *shankhaprakshalana*). *Pranayma* can be practised throughout the year, but do not practise in the heat of the sun or when the body is cold or ill. Practise early in the day, preferably before sunrise, when pollution is at its lowest concentration. You can also practise after sunset, when the air is cool.

Posture

Sit on a folded blanket or cushion in a suitable meditative *asana* for *pranayama*, such as *padmasana* (lotus pose), *siddhasana* (accomplished pose), *swastikasana* (auspicious pose) or *vajrasana* (thunderbolt pose) (see Chapter 8). The posture you choose to sit in should allow you to keep your back erect from the base of the spine to the neck and you should be able to sit comfortably and relaxed with your eyes closed.

Precautions

Do not practise *asanas* immediately after *pranayama*. Relax after strenuous *asana* practise before practising *pranayama*.

Do not practise *pranayama* immediately after meals; allow at least four hours after eating. If you are hungry, just eat a small snack or drink. You can eat half an hour after *pranayama*.

When practising *pranayama* do not force, strain or breathe in jerky movements. Do not struggle to restrain the breath after inhalation or exhalation. If you feel any adverse symptoms, then stop your practice immediately and rest.

If you have practised *pranayama* incorrectly you can do *viparita karani mudra* (see chapter 4), and hold for as long as comfortable, breathing normally. If you feel that too much heat has been generated in the body due to *pranayama*, then stop your practice, apply vegetable oil to the body, head and soles of the feet by massage. A little later, take a hot bath and then lie in *shavasana* (yoga relaxation pose) for 20 minutes to relax.

Women should avoid *kapalabhati* and *bhastrika* (bellows breath) during pregnancy. A long retention of the breath should also be avoided after full exhalation (*bahya kumbhaka*) with *uddiyana bandha*. However, the following *pranayamas* can be practised, and will give benefit: *nadi shuddhi* (alternate nostril breathing), *surya bhedana*, *chandra bhedana*, *viloma pranayama* and *ujjayi pranayama*.

It is safe to practise *pranayama* during the menstrual period, but avoid *uddiyana bandha* (abdominal contraction).

PREPARATION

Before commencing *pranayama* practice, cleanse the nostrils with the *jala neti* technique (see Chapter 4); this also helps to equalize the flow of breath in each nostril. One can also cleanse the nostrils and strengthen the mucous membrane with the technique of *sutra neti* (see chapter 4).

When you have cleansed the nostrils and made sure that all the water has been drained from the nasal passages, it is good to do a few preliminary warm-up exercises to open the chest and lungs to facilitate good breathing. The following is a useful exercise for the lungs.

1 Stand with your feet together with your arms down by your sides. Slowly take a long, deep inhalation as you slowly raise your arms above your head. Stretch right up onto your toes and pull your shoulders back as you stretch your arms up above your head. Then as you exhale, slowly lower your arms back down to your sides. Repeat five times.
2 Stand with the feet hip-width apart and inhale as you raise your arms above your head. Keep your arms straight, but with your hands and wrists relaxed. Exhale as you rotate your arms forward in a wide circle. Imagine yourself as a windmill, and your arms as the turning sails. Breathe deeply and slowly to open the lobes of the lungs. As you raise your arms, inhale and as you lower them, exhale. Practise the forward motion of the arms for five rounds then change direction and rotate them back, pulling your shoulders back as you do so.

You can also practise a few yoga postures that help to open the chest and expand the lungs, such as *ustrasana* (camel pose) *chakrasana* (wheel pose -- see chapter 4) and *matsyasana* (fish pose). These all help to increase the flexibility of the rib cage and the expansion of the lungs.

Ustrasana (camel pose)

Method:
1 Kneel with your thighs at a right angle to the floor. Keep the knees and feet together, and your trunk upright. Place your hands on your hips. Inhale, contract your buttock muscles and raise your hips and trunk.
2 Exhale and arch your back, pushing the pelvis and lumbar region of the spine forwards. Keep your shoulders back and extend your neck.
3 Take each hand back in turn to hold your heels with the palms on the soles, fingers toward the toes. Carefully bend your head back. Hold the pose for ten seconds, gradually increasing to one minute.
4 Inhale. Slowly and carefully raise your trunk up by placing your hands on your hips and contracting your buttocks. Then relax.

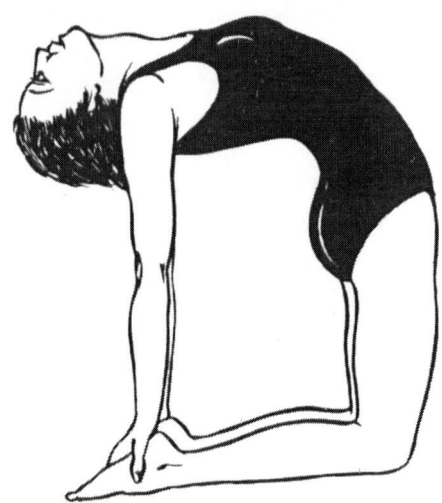

Figure 18 *Ustrasana* (camel pose)

Benefits:
- Opens the chest.
- Gives flexibility to the spine.
- Stimulates digestion.
- Strengthens the lungs and reproductive glands.

Another good posture for preparing the respiration for *pranayama* is *padadirasana* (breath balancing pose). Sit in *vajrasana*, cross your arms and place your hands under your armpits, with the thumbs pointing upwards. With a little pressure, press your fingers against your armpits. Close your eyes and concentrate on the point between the eyebrows. Breathe slowly and rhythmically, with awareness on the breath.

This posture is most beneficial when held for at least ten minutes. It can be practised at any time, even after meals. It keeps both nostrils open, relieving discomfort from blocked nasal passages.

The following breathing exercises are best practised before the *pranayama* session, after opening the lungs.

Cleansing Breath: Exercise 1

Sit in *vajrasana* with your hands resting on your knees, palms down. Inhale a complete yogic breath (see pages 197–9) and hold it for a few seconds. Then pucker your lips and exhale vigorously through them in a series of short, sharp exhalations as you slowly lower your trunk and forehead to the floor. Relax, while holding your breath out for a few seconds, then slowly raise your head and trunk back up while slowly breathing in through the nostrils. Practise three times.

This breath is very beneficial for ventilating and cleansing the lungs. It stimulates the cells and gives a good tone to the respiratory organs. It eliminates carbon dioxide from the system.

Cleansing Breath: Exercise 2

Stand with your feet together, arms relaxed by your sides. Take a complete yogic breath, then with your lips puckered, 'whoosh' the breath out powerfully as you slowly bend at the knees to bring your fingers to the floor. While crouching down, hold your breath out for a few seconds, then slowly breathe in through your nostrils as you stand up. Your arms and back should be kept straight but relaxed throughout the practice. Repeat up to ten times.

This breath cleanses the system of carbon dioxide very quickly. It stimulates the expansion of the blood vessels and the blood pressure falls.

But beware: it should *not* be practised by those with heart problems or problems with blood pressure.

Cleansing Breath for the Nasal Passages and Sinuses

1 Sit in a comfortable posture with your spine straight and your body relaxed.
2 Slowly inhale through both nostrils, hold the breath for two or three seconds, then pucker your lips and exhale all the air from your lungs with a series of dynamic exhalations, like a bellows action.
3 Inhale through your left nostril, closing the right nostril with your right thumb, resting your index and second fingers at the point between your eyebrows.
4 Hold your breath for two or three seconds, then close your left nostril with the third finger of your right hand and exhale through your right nostril, with a series of short, sharp exhalations.
5 Now repeat this process, inhaling through the right nostril and then through both nostrils again.
6 Practise this cleansing breath for one week, starting with one round on the first day, two rounds on the second, three on the third day, and so on.

This cleansing breath is an atomising breath that expels any waste matter or toxins from the nasal passages and sinuses. It is very beneficial for those suffering from congestion in the head.

Prana Mudra (For Awakening the Pranic Energy)

Sit in a comfortable meditative *asana*, close your eyes and relax your body. Place your hands, palms up, in your lap, with the left hand on top of the right. There are six stages, as follows.

1 Emptying the lungs

Exhale deeply, contracting the abdominal muscles, squeezing as much air out of the lungs as possible. Then perform *mulabandha* (see chapter 4) with the breath held out.

2 Starting inhalation to *manipura chakra*
Release *mulabandha* and inhale through both nostrils slowly and deeply, visualizing the breath as a pure white light ascending within the *sushumna nadi*. Simultaneously raise both hands so that the palms and fingers are pointing to your navel. As you inhale focus your awareness at the *manipura chakra* (solar plexus centre) and draw the *prana* up to it from the *muladhara chakra*.

3 Inhalation from *manipura* to *anahata chakra*
Continue inhaling, moving your hands up with the inhaling breath until they are in front of the heart (*anahata chakra*), expanding the chest and filling the upper lungs with air.

4 Inhalation from *anahata* to *vishuddhi* and *ajna chakras*
In the last step of this inhalation, continue inhaling, raising your rib cage under your collarbones to fill the upper lobes of your lungs with air. Simultaneously raise your hands so that they pass in front of your throat (*vishuddhi*) and eyebrow (*ajna*) chakras. Feel the *prana* being drawn up through these chakras.

5 Internal breath retention
Retain the breath and keeping your hands at the level of your ears, stretch your arms out to the side, bent at the elbows and with the palms facing upwards. Now concentrate on the crown chakra (*sahasrara*), visualizing pure white light energy pouring down into you. Feel your entire being radiating with this soothing white light. It surrounds your whole body, then it gradually expands and encompasses the room or area you are in. It continues to expand throughout the whole country, then the whole world, radiating love and peace to all beings. Retain the breath and this feeling for as long as is comfortably possible, without straining the lungs.

6 Exhalation down through the chakras
The exhalation begins in reverse order – exhaling from the top of the lungs first (chest, diaphragm, abdomen). As you exhale, pass your hands simultaneously down in front of the chakras, visualizing the breath as a pure white light descending through the chakras in the *sushumna nadi*.

At the end of the exhalation concentrate on the *muladhara chakra* and repeat steps 2–6.

Practise a minimum of five rounds.

This practice recharges and revitalizes the body and brings peace and serenity to the mind.

Stimulating and Cleansing the Lung Cells

This is a very stimulating breathing exercise which activates the air cells in the lungs and invigorates the whole body.

1. Stand with your feet hip-width apart.
2. Inhale with a long, slow, deep breath (complete yogic breath – see pages 197–9) and simultaneously tap all over your chest with your fingertips.
3. Retain the breath and pat all over your chest with the palms of your hands.
4. Pucker your lips and exhale powerfully, blowing or 'whooshing' the breath out through your mouth. Extend your arms out in front of you and lean forward with your head down as you exhale.
5. Hold your breath out while leaning forward in the standing position for as long as is comfortable, then slowly inhale through both nostrils as you slowly come back to the upright position.

Caution: If you feel dizzy then discontinue the practice. In the beginning you may do so, but with careful practice you will overcome the dizziness.

Swara Yoga

The Sanskrit word *swara* is from the root *swar*, 'to sound'. *Swara* basically means 'air inhaled through the nostrils'. Swara Yoga is the ancient science of studying the flow of *prana*, and is also known as Swarodaya and Swara Vijnana.

The Swara yogis of India studying this science experimented and made great detailed correlations between the way the breath flowed and various physiological and psychological states. They produced detailed lists of examples, some of which are represented in the table below. The figures represent the various distances from the nose that the exhalation of air can be felt during a person's different activities and moods. The length of the breath is mentioned in the classical yoga treatise, the *Gheranda Samhita*. The body of *vayu* (air) is 96 digits (6 feet) in standard length.

Normal state	–	6 digits (4½ inches)
During emotion	–	12 digits (9 inches)
During singing	–	16 digits (12 inches)
While eating	–	20 digits (15 inches)
While walking	–	24 digits (18 inches)
During sleeping	–	30 digits (22 inches)
During sexual intercourse	–	36 digits (27 inches)
During physical exercise	–	over 36 digits.

(Note: One digit equals ¼ inch)

You can measure your own breath by moistening the back of your hand and holding it under your nostrils. As you exhale you will feel the air blowing on to your skin. Then measure the length of your breath from hand to nostrils.

SWARA YOGA AND LONGEVITY

Yogis have stated that a person who breathes shallowly in short, sharp gasps is likely to reduce his or her lifespan, compared with a person who breathes slowly and deeply. So sure were they of this principle that they measured a person's lifespan, not in years but by the number of breaths. They considered that each individual is allocated a fixed number of breaths in their lifetime, with the number varying from person to person. Therefore if a person breathes slowly and deeply, they not only gain more vitality but they also optimize their experience of life.

The ancient yogis who lived in the forests of India, or in secluded hill or mountain regions, had intimate contact with nature all around them. In this natural environment they were able to study the wild animals in great detail. They discovered that animals with a slow breathing rate, such as snakes, crocodiles, elephants and tortoises, have a long lifespan. Conversely, they noticed that animals with a fast breathing rate, such as birds, cats, dogs and rabbits, live only for a few years. It was from this observation that they realized the importance of slow breathing.

It is also interesting to note that the respiration is directly related to the heartbeat. Slow respiration occurs with a slow-beating heart, which is conducive to a long lifespan. For example, a whale's heart beats about

16 times a minute, and an elephant's approximately 25. Both these animals are renowned for their long lifespans. A mouse's heart, on the other hand beats approximately 1,000 times a minute, and it lives a short life.

It is said by the yogis that a normal person breathes 21,000 breaths a day and in comparison to some of his or her friends in the animal kingdom, lives a relatively short life.

There have been, and there still are, many great yogis who have lived or are living very long lives; their vital endurance is remarkably increased by the practice of yoga, *pranayama* and meditation. Through their yogic practices and attunement with God and the laws of Nature, they have mastery and control over the life-force of the body, attaining the power to shed the physical body at will or to retain it for an indefinite period of time.

Among such masters of yoga are Lokanath Brahmachari, who lived for 166 years and Shivapuri Baba, the great yogi and master of alchemy, who died in 1963 at the age of 137 years. Swami Rama of the Himalayan International Institute of Yoga Science and Philosophy in Pennsylvania, USA, met an ageless yogi at the 1974 Kumbha Mela (a great spiritual fair held every 12 years in India). This yogi's name is Devraha Baba and he is said to be over 150 years old. It was discovered that he eats only fruits and vegetables, and practises certain aspects of yoga regularly.

Paramhansa Yogananda stated in his *Autobiography of a Yogi* that Lahiri Mahasaya had a very famous friend called Swami Trailanga, who was reputed to be over 300 years old. But the most amazing of them all must be the divine Mahavatar Babaji of the Himalayas, the guru of Lahiri Mahasaya and the Paramguru of Paramhansa Yogananda. Babaji, the 'divine Yogi Avatara' is eternal, with an immortal body. He has miraculous powers and control over time, decay and death. He can materialize or de-materialize his physical body at will. His undecaying body requires no food and he appears to his spiritually advanced disciples in the Himalayas from time to time. There have been disciples, in this lifetime, who have seen him. You can read more about Babaji in Paramhansa Yogananda's inspiring book, *Autobiography of A Yogi*.

By understanding and experience in the knowledge and practice of Swara Yoga, *pranayama*, *kriyas*, *asanas*, deep meditation and deep selfless love for God and mankind one can prevent disease, preserve health and youth, and promote longevity.

The Flow of Breath (*Prana*)

A very interesting and observable phenomenon of Swara Yoga is that the flow of air through the nostrils is very rarely equal. This again can be experienced and tested by moistening the back of the hand and breathing on it, to feel in which nostril the air is flowing more predominantly, or to feel if they are flowing equally.

During the course of a day, the flow of air or *prana* is dominantly flowing in either the left nostril (*ida nadi*) or the right (*pingala nadi*), or evenly flowing through both (*sushumna nadi*).

When the breath and the *nadis* are functioning normally, the breath flow alternates between the left and the right nostril every two hours. Physiologically this occurs because of a mild swelling and expansion of the tissue covering the nasal turbinates and the septum within one of the nostrils. This results in one nostril gradually becoming obstructed, which decreases the flow of air in that nostril, which in turn causes a shift in the flow of air to the opposite nostril.

During the few minutes when nostril dominance is changing, the air flows more evenly through both. This alternation of the natural breath flow in each nostril is due to biological changes caused by the mind's fluctuating mental states, and to environmental and lunar influences.

The Swara yogis discovered through their studies of healthy, balanced people during the waxing and waning of the moon, that the breath flow in the nostrils was affected by the lunar energies. They observed that at sunrise, the breath flow rises in the left nostril (*ida nadi*) on the first lunar day when the moon is waxing (bright fortnight). Then the breath flow alternates at the end of each hour, moving from the left nostril (*ida nadi*) to the right (*pingala nadi*). The breath flow then continues alternating from one nostril to the other every hour for three days. On the fourth day at sunrise the breath flow rises in the right nostril (*pingala nadi*).

At sunrise, on the first lunar day, when the moon is waning (dark fortnight), the breath flow is reversed and begins rising in the right nostril (*pingala nadi*).

When the breath flow is dominant in the right nostril a person is more inclined to physical action than to thinking or intellectual pursuits. This is because the right nostril is associated with the sun current, warmth, heat, action and the physical. Left-brain activity becomes dominant.

The inclination to action is reversed when the left nostril is dominant, producing a calmer state of mind. The cool moon current influences the right-brain tendencies of introspection, mental creativity and creative imagination.

This flow of breath is constantly alternating from one nostril to the other approximately every one and three quarters to two hours. Apparently this is a natural rhythm, but it can change with our fluctuating mental and emotional states, activities, disease, stress and the unbalancing of our daily routines. This natural rhythmic cycle is necessary for balancing the mind and body. Without this balance, serious harm can occur. If the breath were to flow in only one nostril for 24 hours or more, then one would become very ill – there would be an imbalance.

When the breath is flowing equally through both nostrils then the *sushumna* (the central *nadi*) functions. In this balanced state, the mental processes are clear and calm; the body and the breath are calm and steady. Meditation and contemplation become effortless when the breath is flowing in the *sushumna*. But when either the mind or breath becomes restless, this brings about a disturbance in the balance of the breath flow in the *nadis*.

If one is to be successful in meditation then *sushumna* must be flowing. If *pingala* flows the body will be restless; if *ida* flows, thoughts will distract you from meditating.

How to Balance and Change The Flow

There are various methods for changing the flow of breath in the *nadis*. If you wish to change the flow from the right nostril to the left, you can use any of the following methods. To change from the left to the right, reverse the process.

- Lie down on your right side for ten minutes. It is traditional for yogis to sleep on their right side with the left nostril flow (*ida*) open for a calm, relaxing sleep. If the *pingala* flows predominantly at night you may become restless and find it difficult to sleep.
- Squeeze your left hand under your right arm, so that the fingers are pressing into the armpit.

PRANAYAMA 189

- Close off your right nostril with a piece of cotton wool for a few minutes, until the flow changes to the left nostril.
- Practise *nauli kriya* (see chapter 4).
- Practise *kechari mudra* (see chapter 4).
- Use will-power to change the flow.
- To balance the *nadis* by changing the flow to the *sushumna*, concentrate at the point between the eyebrows (the spiritual eye), or concentrate on any one of the chakras. When your body is steady and your spine straight, seated in *asana*, with your mind concentrated and quiet, then your *sushumna* functions.
- Practise *padadirasana* (see page 181) to keep the flow even in both nostrils.

PURIFICATION OF THE *NADIS* THROUGH *PRANAYAMA*

The *Nadis*

The *nadis* are a network of astral nerves situated throughout the astral body. The two main *nadis* are the *ida* and the *pingala*. The *ida* and the *pingala* correspond to the left and right sympathetic nerve cords in the physical body. Through these astral tubes flows the vital life-force, called *prana*. In between these two nadis is the *sushumna nadi*, which is the most important of all the *nadis*. The *sushumna nadi* is the central channel into which the yogi tries to direct the pranic flow, so as to stimulate and awaken the *kundalini shakti* (a force of energy).

Throughout the subtle or astral body there are about 72,000 *nadis* which circulate *prana* throughout the body. In the *Brihadaranyaka Upanishad*, a Vedic scripture, which is the oldest of the *Upanishads*, dating from about 800 BC, it says that the *nadis* are as fine as a hair split into 1,000.

The *nadis'* source, which is egg-shaped and called *kanda*, is located between the anus and the root of the genitals, just above the *muladhara chakra*. This is also the junction of the *sushumna* and the *muladhara chakra*. From *kanda* the *nadis* distribute *prana* all over the body.

One way of purifying the *nadis* is to practise the *shatkarmas* (see chapter 4), but some Westerners find these rather strenuous and tiring.

Another way is to practise the following purification exercises in the exact order as given:

1 *nadi shuddhi* (alternate nostril breathing)
2 *kapalabhati* (skull-shining breathing)
3 *agni sara dhauti* (fire wash)
4 *ashwini mudra* (horse mudra)

Practise these techniques for a period of three months before beginning your *pranayama* programme. They will purify the *nadis* and strengthen and purify the nerves of the physical body. The last three techniques are explained in chapter 4. The following is the technique for *nadi shuddhi*.

Nadi Shuddhi: Alternate Nostril Breathing

This *pranayama* is also known as *anuloma-viloma* when breath retention is added.

This nerve-purifying breathing also maintains an equilibrium in the catabolic and anabolic processes in the body. It purifies the blood and the brain cells. It has a soothing effect on the nervous system.

For the yogi it is usual to make the breath flow in each nostril exactly the same. When the flow of air is equal in each nostril, then the flow in the *ida* and *pingala nadis* is also the same – they become balanced. Under these balanced conditions, *prana* begins to flow in the central main *nadi* (*sushumna*).

1 Begin by sitting comfortably in *asana*, with the head, neck and spine in a straight line. Keep the body still and relaxed.
2 Place your left hand on your left knee, relaxed, and raise the right hand to your face. Make the *vishnu mudra* by folding down your index and middle fingers.
3 Exhale through both nostrils. Then close your right nostril with your thumb and inhale slowly and deeply through your left nostril.
4 Close your left nostril with your third and fourth fingers, release your thumb and exhale through your right nostril.
5 Inhale through your right nostril, then close it with your thumb and exhale through your left nostril.

	1: 2: 2 RATIO *Ratios for* *Beginners*			1: 4: 2 RATIO *Ratios for the* *Advanced*		
	IN	HOLD	OUT	IN	HOLD	OUT
Stage 1	4:	8:	8	4:	16:	8
Stage 2	5:	10:	10	5:	20:	10
Stage 3	6:	12:	12	6:	24:	12
Stage 4	7:	14:	14	7:	28:	14
Stage 5	8:	16:	16	8:	32:	16

This completes one round. To start with, practise only ten rounds, then gradually increase to 40 rounds by increasing by one round each week.

The relative measures of breath inhalation (*purak*), retention (*kumbak*) and exhalation (*rechak*) are:

- 1: 2: 2 for beginners who are advised to follow this ratio for a few months before taking up the advanced ratio.
- 1: 4: 2 for advanced students of *pranayama*

For beginners this means that the breath retention is twice that of the inhalation, and the period of exhalation is the same as that of the retention. For advanced students it means that the breath retention is four times that of the inhalation, and the period of exhalation is twice that of the inhalation.

The minimum starting proportion for a beginner is 4: 8: 8 (if this is difficult then start from 2: 4: 4). After having practised this ratio for one month, then increase the ratio to 5: 10: 10. Then increase gradually until you reach 8: 16: 16. On no account should you increase this proportion until you are able to practise it with comfort and ease. You must *never* force or strain the breath and lungs; to do so could cause damage to the physical body. If you are not sure then consult a qualified teacher who practises *pranayama*.

As you progress with these ratios, you will be able to change to the advanced ratio of 1: 4: 2, gradually working up to 8: 32: 16, which could take all of two years' practice to reach. A student who wants to go beyond this limit is advised to seek personal instruction from a competent teacher of *pranayama*.

Commence with three rounds, gradually increasing to 20. Increase the proportionate ratios and the number of rounds very slowly.

When the breath is retained for longer than ten seconds, then it is important to hold *jalandhara bandha* (chin lock). See chapter 4 for the technique.

Nadi Shuddhi Exercises for Beginners

1 Practise ten rounds of inhaling and exhaling through the left nostril. Then repeat ten rounds of inhaling and exhaling through the right nostril. (Simple breathing – no ratio).
2 Practise ten rounds of inhaling through the left nostril, then exhaling through the right. Repeat ten rounds of inhaling through the right nostril and exhaling through the left (Simple breathing – no ratio).
3 Practise five rounds of inhaling through the left nostril, holding the breath for five seconds, and exhaling through the right nostril.
4 Practise five rounds of inhaling through the right nostril, holding the breath for five seconds, and exhaling through the left nostril.
5 Inhale through the left nostril. Hold the breath inside. Exhale through the right nostril, and retain the breath outside. Breathe in through the right nostril. Retain the breath inside. Exhale through the left nostril and retain the breath outside. Practise this simple breathing without a proportionate ratio for five rounds.

This uses internal and external breath retention *antaranga kumbhaka* and *bahiranga kumbhaka*. The starting ratio for this is 1 : 4 : 2 : 2, and as in the other exercises, it should be increased gradually over a period of time.

Advanced *Nadi Shuddhi*

The following three practices must only be done by those who have advanced sufficiently to be able to hold the breath comfortably with the use of *bandhas* for one minute. One needs to have practised the basic

PRANAYAMA 193

pranayamas using proportionate ratios for at least one year, and be experienced in applying the *bandhas* when retaining the breath internally and externally.

The following practices use the ratio, 16: 64: 32.

First *pranayama*

1 Sit in the lotus posture (*padmasana*) or *siddhasana* and meditate on the element of air (*vayu*), which is a smoky colour.
2 Inhale through the left nostril and mentally repeat the *bija mantra yam* as you breathe in for a count of 16 seconds.
3 Hold your breath until you have mentally repeated the *yam* 64 times.
4 Exhale through the right nostril, until you have mentally repeated *yam* 32 times.

Second *pranayama*

1 Sit in *padmasana* or *siddhasana* and meditate on the element of fire (*agni*).
2 Inhale through your right nostril, mentally repeating 16 times with the breath, the *agni bija mantra ram*.
3 Hold your breath until you have mentally repeated *ram* 64 times.
4 Exhale through your left nostril until you have mentally repeated *ram* 32 times.

Third *pranayama*

1 Sit in *padmasana* or *siddhasana* with your inner attention focused at the spiritual eye, the point between the eyebrows.
2 Inhale through your left nostril, mentally repeating the *bija mantra tham* with the breath 16 times.
3 Hold your breath until you have mentally repeated the *tham* 64 times. Simultaneously, visualize the cool nectar from the moon flowing through all the vessels and *nadis* of your body, purifying them.
4 Exhale through your right nostril, mentally repeating the earth element (*prithvi*) *bija mantra lam*, 32 times.

Four Different Methods of Breathing

In yoga the breathing process is classified into four general methods:

- abdominal or diaphragmatic or low breathing
- intercostal or middle breathing
- clavicular or upper breathing
- complete yogic breathing (which is a combination of low, middle and upper breathing)

Abdominal breathing is associated with the movement of the diaphragm and the outer wall of the abdomen. When relaxed the diaphragm muscle arches upwards like a parachute into the chest region. During inhalation the diaphragm muscle is flattened from a dome shape to a disc shape, as it moves downwards. This compresses the abdominal organs and eventually pushes the front wall, the navel, of the abdomen outwards. This movement enlarges the chest cavity downwards and allows the diaphragm to move upwards again, to reduce the volume in the chest cavity, which causes exhalation.

This form of breathing is physiologically the most efficient because it draws in the greatest amount of air for the least amount of muscular effort.

In *Intercostal breathing* the movement of the ribs is brought into play. During expansion of the ribcage outwards and upwards by muscular contraction, the lungs are allowed to expand. This results in air being drawn down into them from the front side and inhalation taking place. The intercostal muscles control the movements of the ribs – when they are relaxed, then the ribs move downwards and inwards. This movement compresses the lungs and exhalation takes place.

In *Clavicular breathing*, inhalation and deflation of the lungs is achieved by raising the upper ribs, shoulders and collarbones (clavicles). This method requires maximum effort to obtain minimum benefit. Very little air is inhaled and exhaled, since this movement cannot change the volume of the chest cavity very much. Upper breathing is common in Western society, owing to the modern lifestyles we have adopted, particularly in the cities and large towns where we are more open to stressful conditions – pollution, noise, overheated and unventilated rooms and offices, badly designed chairs and other people's smoke. We get into a state of anxiety or we immobilize our diaphragm in an attempt to contain our fears of aggression and other deep emotional feelings, causing us to breathe shallowly in the upper chest.

Complete yogic breathing combines all the above modes of breathing into one complete harmonious movement. In that form of respiration the entire respiratory system is brought into use – all the respiratory muscles including the internal and external intercostals and abdominal muscles; the ribcage; every part of the lungs and their air cells; and the diaphragm. It is this type of breathing that we are interested in developing, since only yogic breathing can give the maximum inhalation and exhalation of breath.

COMPLETE YOGIC BREATH PRACTISED IN SECTIONS

The purpose of this practice is to make you aware of the three different types of respiration, and to incorporate them into the complete yogic breath. It also corrects shallow breathing and calms the mind.

For the practice of these exercises sit in a comfortable posture, either cross-legged or in *vajrasana*, with the spine straight in a warm but well-ventilated room. All breathing should be performed through the nostrils and not through the mouth.

Abdominal Breathing (*Adham Pranayama*)

1 Place the palms of your hands lightly on your abdomen. This is to make you aware of the movement in your abdomen as the air is breathed in and out of the lowest lobes of your lungs. Breathe out slowly and completely, remembering that it is the movement of your diaphragm that is responsible for your abdominal breathing. As you exhale, feel your abdomen contract; your navel will move toward the spine. At the end of exhalation the diaphragm will be totally relaxed and will be doming or parachuting upwards into the chest cavity.
2 Now hold your breath for one or two seconds.
3 Inhale, without expanding your chest or moving your shoulders. Feel your abdomen expand, the navel moving upwards. The breathing should be deep and slow. At the end of the inhalation your diaphragm

will be bowing in the direction of the abdomen and your navel will be at its highest point.
4 Hold the breath for one or two seconds.
5 Exhale again, slowly and completely. At the end of the exhalation your abdomen will be contracted. Hold the breath for a short time, inhale and then repeat the whole process twice more.
6 Now move your hands around to your back, so that your palms are resting on your lower back, with the fingers pointing towards the spine. Concentrate your mind on the movement of the lungs beneath your hands as you breathe. Repeat the same breathing process as you did for the abdomen three times.

Middle or Intercostal Breathing (*Madhyam Pranayama*)

In this practice the idea is to breathe by utilizing the movement of the ribcage. Throughout this practice try not to move the abdomen; this is achieved by slightly contracting the abdominal muscles.

1 Place your palms either side of the middle ribcage, so that the fingers of each hand are pointing towards each other. This is to feel the expansion and contraction of the ribs. The intercostals (the muscles between the ribs) swing the ribs upwards and forwards, increasing the diameter of the chest and expanding the lungs, while the internal intercostals pull the ribs down, causing a reduction in lung volume.
2 Breathe in slowly by expanding the ribcage outwards and upwards. You will find it impossible to breathe deeply because of the limitation on the maximum expansion of the chest.
3 At the end of the inhalation, hold your breath for one or two seconds.
4 Slowly exhale by contracting the chest downwards and inwards. Keep the abdomen slightly contracted, but without strain.
5 Breathe in slowly. Repeat the whole process twice more.
6 Then place your hands behind the mid-area of your back, opposite to where you had your hands placed on your front. Again, concentrate and breathe into the middle back area for three rounds.

Upper or Clavicular Breathing (*Adhyam Pranayama*)

In this practice try not to expand or contract your abdomen or chest – not easy to do.

1 Place both palms on your upper chest, above your breasts, so that you can determine whether your chest is moving or not, while trying not to contract the muscles of your abdomen.
2 Inhale by drawing your collarbones and shoulders towards your chin. You may find this difficult at first, but persevere. A good method is to inhale and exhale with a sniffing action, which automatically induces upper breathing.
3 Exhale by letting your shoulders and collarbones move away from your chin.
4 Practise this technique twice more.
5 Then place your hands on your hips, keeping your armpits open. With concentration breathe into the side high lobes of the lungs, so that you feel the movement and breath under the armpits.
6 Repeat this process twice more, then raise your arms over your shoulders, and over the higher lobes of the lungs. Breathe deeply and slowly into this area three times with concentration.

The Complete Yogic Breath Technique

The combination of the three types of breathing – low, middle and upper – takes the optimum volume of air into the lungs and expels the maximum amount of carbon dioxide.

1 Breathe out deeply, contracting the abdomen to squeeze all the air from the lungs.
2 Inhale slowly, keeping the lower part of the abdomen contracted, while expanding the part above the navel slightly. The reason for this is that if you push the lower abdomen out, you are likely to acquire a pot belly due to the abdominal organs moving down and forward.
3 At the end of the upper abdomen expansion, start to expand your chest and ribcage outwards and upwards. Continue drawing the

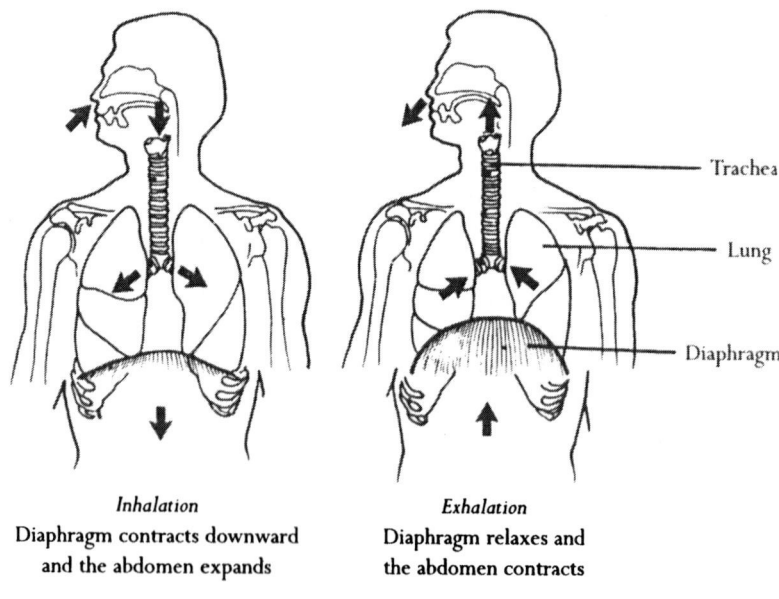

Figure 19 *Yogic Breathing*

breath upwards into the higher lobes of your lungs by raising your collarbones and shoulders towards your head. Your lungs should now be completely filled with air.

4 Hold your breath in for a few seconds, with the head forward in *jalandhara bandha* (see chapter 4). This is practised by gently dropping the head forward so that the chin rests in the notch between the collarbones. Do not strain or force your neck into the position, but keep the neck and throat muscles soft and relaxed. Move your chest upwards to meet your chin as you bring it down, then you will not strain the neck or throat. Only hold *jalandhara bandha* for a few seconds or for as long as is comfortable while holding the breath.

5 Release the chin lock by raising your head and begin to exhale, first relaxing your collarbones and shoulders. Then allow your chest to move first downwards and then inwards. After this allow the

abdomen to contract. Do not strain but try to empty your lungs as much as possible, squeezing all the air out by drawing the abdominal wall closer to the spine.
6 Hold your breath out for a few seconds. This completes one round of yogic breathing. Now take a few normal breaths, then practise another five rounds.

The whole movement should be one continuous movement, each phase of breathing merging into the next, without there being any obvious transition point. There should be no strain or jerky movements with the body or breath. The body should remain relaxed throughout the practice. With practice you will find that the whole process will occur naturally with no undue effort.

The reason for practising *jalandhara bandha* (chin lock) is to retain the pressure of the air within the lungs so as to reduce any pressure in the brain and regulate the flow of blood and *prana* to the head, heart and thyroid glands in the throat.

This practice develops good healthy lung tissues which resist germs, making you much less susceptible to disease. The blood receives plenty of oxygen and every organ of the body is nourished by it. Digestion and assimilation are improved, and bodily energy and vigour are increased. The nervous system and the brain benefit through the blood being properly oxygenated, making them more efficient instruments for generating, storing and transmitting the nerve currents. Clarity of thought is improved.

To develop yogic breathing as an automatic and normal function of the body, develop the habit of consciously breathing yogically for a few minutes whenever you can throughout the day. If you feel tired, depressed, angry or anxious, then become centred within yourself and sit down, or if possible lie down, and practise yogic breathing. Breathe deeply and slowly with your concentration on the breath. Feel that you are inhaling not just air, but joy, peace, strength, courage or whatever positive quality you want especially to affirm. As you exhale, breathe away any negative qualities that your mind may be holding on to. Then your mind will become calm and revitalized.

HAND *MUDRAS* FOR CONTROLLING THE BREATH

The hand *mudras* covered in this section control the physical functions of the breathing. The *mudra* achieves this by controlling the mind-brain processes and the functions within the nervous system by uniting various nerve terminals of the sympathetic and parasympathetic nervous systems.

In chapter 4, we discussed the main *mudras*, such as *yoni mudra* in which the state of *pratyahara* (sense withdrawal) is brought about by the pressure of the fingers on the face, upon the vagus and the facial nerves, which are brought together in a closed circuit. In *yoni mudra*, which was also discussed in chapter 4, the hands are united with the feet, which causes the vagus nerve system to be close-circuited with the cerebrospinal nerves.

When the hands are placed together palm to palm, as in the praying gesture of the Christians, Jews and Hindus, the cranial nerve circuits in the head and the upper part of the body in the pneumogastric or vagus nerve system are united together.

The right lung is divided into three separate compartments or lobes: the lower abdominal lobe, the middle intracostal lobe and the high clavicular or superior lobe. The left lung has only two lobes: the lower and the higher.

A section of the brain controls each of these lung lobes via the nervous system. By applying the hand *mudras* in certain combinations, each lobe can be inflated and deflated independently of one another. This gives one greater control over the breath and *prana*.

In some of the *pranayama* techniques which follow, we will use five basic hand mudras:

- Chinmaya or jnana mudra. This controls abdominal breathing (*adham pranayama*). Make a circle by joining together the tip of the thumb and the first finger. The other three fingers are kept outstretched and together.
- Chin mudra (the symbol of wisdom). This controls the middle lobes of the lungs (*madhyam pranayama*). Join together the tip of the thumb and the first finger to form a circle. The other three fingers are folded into the palm of the hand, with the tips of the fingers tightly pressed in.

- *Adhi mudra.* This controls the high clavicular or superior lobes of the lungs (*adhyam pranayama*). Fold the thumb into your palm and fold the other fingers over the thumb, clenching them into a fist.
- *Brahma mudra.* This controls complete yogic breathing (*mahat yoga pranayama*) in each of the three parts of the lungs. The hands are clenched into position as in *adhi mudra*, then the knuckles where the fingers join the hand are pressed together, hand to hand, with the fingers turned upwards. The hands in this position are then lowered below the diaphragm, in front of the navel.
- *Shunya mudra* (*shunya* means vacuum or void). This *mudra* keeps a lobe of the lung empty while others are being inflated. Open one palm, with the thumb at a 90-degree angle to the palm. Make sure the fingers are extended and tightly together. Place the hand, palm upward, on the junction of the thigh close in to the body.

VIBHAGA PRANAYAMA: SECTIONAL BREATHING

This practice calms the mind and increases the air intake into the lungs. It harmoniously develops the various parts of the lungs.

1 Sit in *vajrasana*, close your eyes and relax. Place your hands in *chin mudra*, position both hands palms down at the top of your thighs, close to your groin, with the fingers turned inwards. Now inhale from the abdomen, then exhale. Practise six rounds of this breath.
2 Place your hands in *chinmaya mudra*, position both hands at the top of the thighs again. Breathe into the mid-chest lobes of the lungs. The intercostal muscles between the ribs expand and the rib cage opens like an accordion. Inhale and exhale six times.
3 Now position your hands in *adhi mudra* by clenching your fists, with the thumbs inside touching the palms. Place your hands fingers down on your upper thighs close to the groin. Inhale into the upper lobes of your lungs (just below the collarbones), then exhale. Practise this breathing six times.
4 With your hands still in *adhi mudra*, place both hands together in front of the navel, with the knuckles of each hand pressed together and turned upwards in *brahma mudra*. Now inhale a complete yogic breath, combining the three stages of lower, middle and upper

breathing in one long, slow, deep, smooth continuous breath. Then exhale; the breath will empty out first from the lower lungs, then the middle, followed by the upper lungs.

Controlling the Breath with *Shunya Mudra*

1 Sit in *vajrasana*, close your eyes and relax.
2 Place your left hand in any one of the following *mudras*: *chin*, *chinmaya* or *adhi*. The palm should be resting on the top of your left thigh close to your body. Place your right hand in *shunya mudra*, palm upwards on top of the right thigh.
3 Now inhale deeply and you will find that the lobe of the lung on the right side will not be activated; it will remain empty, while the left lobe of the lung indicated by the *mudra* of your left hand will inflate and deflate with the respiration.
4 Reverse the *mudras*, so that you have your left hand in *shunya mudra* and your right hand in *chin*, *chinmaya* or *adhi*. Then breathe in deeply.
5 You can also try controlling the breath in various lobes of the lungs by using *chin*, *chinmaya* or *adhi mudra* with both the left and right hand using different combinations. For example, if you have the left hand in *chin mudra* and the right hand in *adhi mudra* you will get the extraordinary feeling of the breath crossing diagonally from the lower lobe of the left lung to the upper lobe of the right lung as you inhale deeply.

PRANAYAMA TECHNIQUES

SUKHA PRANAYAMA: PLEASANT BREATH

Exercise 1: This is a very simple *pranayama* that even children and convalescents can practise. It simply involves inhaling and exhaling equally through both nostrils, but it is important to make sure that the inhalation is of the same duration as the exhalation. To begin with you can use a metronome or the tick of a clock for counting the breaths.

Practise the following breathing ratios:

INHALE	EXHALE
2	2
3	3
4	4
5	5 (good for people who are always late)
6	6 (good for neurotic and psychotic people)
7	7 (good for introverts)

Exercise 2: *Loma Pranayama*: This is a three-part equal breath ratio: inhale for six, retain for six, exhale for six (6: 6: 6). Practise a minimum of nine rounds every morning and gradually increase to 27 rounds.

Exercise 3: *Viloma Pranayama*: This is also called inverse breathing. Inhale for six, exhale for six, external retention for six (6: 6: 6). Practise nine rounds and gradually increase to 27 rounds. This is good for mothers with a young child. Hold the child and breathe in this ratio. The child will naturally breathe with you.

Exercise 4: *Sukha Purvaka Pranayama*: Inhale for six, retain for six, exhale for six, external retention for six (6: 6: 6: 6).

PANCHA SAHITA PRANAYAMA: THE FIVE-PART-RATIO BREATH

The *pancha sahita pranayama* concentrates on rejuvenating five important body organs – the lungs, liver, digestive organs, elimination organs and heart – using the classical *pranayama anuloma-viloma* over a period of 45 days. It controls the five elements associated with the five body organs and the five pranic flows (*prana vayus*).

The best times to practise this *pranayama* are at sunrise, midday and at sunset.

1. Sit comfortably with your head, neck and spine in a straight line in a meditative *asana*.
2. Practise nine rounds of *anuloma-viloma pranayama* using the proportionate ratio of 4: 16: 8: 4 (to rejuvenate the lungs) three or four times a day, for nine days. The four count is for the inhalation; the sixteen count for the internal breath retention; the eight count for the exhalation and the four count for the external breath retention.

3 On the tenth day, change the breathing ratio to 4: 4: 16: 8 (to rejuvenate the liver). Again, practise three or four times a day, for nine days.
4 Continue with the rejuvenation of the other three organs. To make this clearer use this chart for easy reference.

DAY	BODY ORGAN	Inhale (purak)	Inner Retention (antaranga kumbhaka)	Exhale (rechak)	Outer Retention (bahiranga kumbhaka)
1–9	Lungs	4	16	8	4
10-18	Liver	4	4	16	8
19–27	Digestive Organs	8	4	4	16
28–36	Elimination Organs	16	8	4	4
37–45	Heart	4	16	8	–

This entire *pranayama* routine can be practised once every three months.

Remember to apply *jalandhara bandha* during inner breath retentions of over ten seconds.

BHASTRIKA PRANAYAMA: BELLOWS

The Sanskrit word *bhastrika* means 'bellows'. Just as a blacksmith's bellows blow air vigorously and rapidly to fan the flames of the fire, so in this practice, the practitioner inhales and exhales rapidly in the same way.

This *pranayama* can awaken the *kundalini shakti* if the *nadis* and nervous system are purified.

Within the *sushumna* in the spinal column are three *granthis* (knots). These knots or energy blocks prevent the free movement of the *prana* energy in the *sushumna*.

They are:

- *Brahma granthi* – *muladhara chakra*
- *Vishnu granthi* – *manipura chakra*
- *Rudra granthi* – *ajna chakra*

To free the pranic current and break these knots, one needs to perform *bhastrika pranayama*. When they are broken, the *kundalini* is free to rise gradually toward the *sahasrara chakra* (crown centre), the subtle counterpart of the brain.

1. Sit in a comfortable *asana*, preferably *padmasana* or *siddhasana*, with the spine straight. Relax and close your eyes.
2. Inhale and exhale through both nostrils vigorously and rapidly, so that the expulsions of breath follow one another in rapid succession. This will bring into rapid action both the diaphragm and the entire respiratory apparatus. One rapid inhalation and exhalation completes one *bhastrika* breath.
3. Practise ten breaths, breathing out deeply on the tenth expulsion. Then take a long, slow, deep inhalation through both nostrils.
4. Retain the breath for as long as is comfortable, applying *jalandhara bandha* (chin lock) and *mulabandha* (anal lock) (see chapter 4), with your awareness and concentration on the *kundalini* in the *muladhara chakra*.
5. Release the chin lock, then the anal lock, and exhale slowly.

This completes one round of *bhastrika*. Take a short rest between each round by taking a few normal breaths. As you progress you can gradually increase the number of breaths from ten to 15, 20, 25, 30 and so on up to 120 in each round.

Beginners should start with three to five rounds of ten breaths and gradually increase to a maximum of 30 over a period of months. Advanced students should gradually work up to 120 breaths in each round as a maximum. The rounds can be increased from 20 in the morning to 20 in the evening. The breath retention (*kumbhaka*) can also gradually be increased, but with care and proper guidance from a qualified and experienced teacher of *pranayama*.

This practice increases the supply of blood to the brain, tones the entire nervous system, increases the gastric fire and gives warmth to the body. It helps to cure diseases of the lungs, awakens *kundalini*, activates the *ajna* and *sahasrara chakras* and induces tranquillity to the mind.

However, people with high blood pressure, vertigo or heart ailments should not practise it, and beginners should practise cautiously and seek expert guidance, for this is a powerful *pranayama*.

Alternate Nostril *Bhastrika* (Variation 1)

1. Sit in *vajrasana* and inhale deeply through both nostrils, as you raise your arms above your head and circle them three times while holding the breath. Keep your chest open and lower the left arm, so that you rest your left hand with the palm upwards in your lap.
2. Place the index finger and second finger of your right hand at the point between the eyebrows, and close your left nostril with your third finger. Exhale slowly and deeply through your right nostril, then take a short inhalation through the same nostril and begin the *bhastrika* breathing in the right nostril for ten breaths.
3. On the tenth expulsion, hold the breath out, and apply the three *bandhas*: *jalandhara*, *uddiyana* and then *mula* (see chapter 4). Hold it for as long as is comfortable, without strain. Then release *mulabandha* first, then *uddiyana*, followed by *jalandhara*.
4. Inhale slowly and deeply through the right nostril and hold the breath in for as long as is comfortable, applying the chin lock and anal lock. Release the locks and exhale through the right nostril.
5. Return to normal breathing. This completes one round. Take a short rest before starting steps 1–4 with the left nostril.

The number of rounds and breaths are the same as for the last exercise.

Alternate Nostril *Bhastrika* (Variation 2)

1. Sit upright in a comfortable *asana*, relax and close your eyes.
2. Place your hands in *vishnu mudra* (the thumb of the right hand is used to close the right nostril and direct the *pingala* energies. The third and fourth fingers are used to close the left nostril and direct the *ida* energies).
3. Inhale through the left nostril, exhale through the right nostril, inhale through the right, exhale through the left, inhale through the left and so on. Start slowly at first, then begin to speed the movements up, so that the hand movements which are alternating the breath rapidly in each nostril are synchronized with the breath.

Note: *Bhastrika pranayama* is best practised after *nadi shuddhi* (see pages 190–3).

Bhastrika and Kapalabhati

Kapalabhati is one of the purification exercises (*shatkarmas*) described in chapter 4. The difference between *bhastrika* and *kapalabhati* is that in *bhastrika* the breath is retained at the end of each round with the three *bandhas* to unite the *prana* and *apana*. In *kapalabhati* there is no breath retention.

Kapalabhati also differs in that the inhalation is long and mild, and the exhalation is forceful and rapid, whereas in *bhastrika*, the inhalation is as rapid as the exhalation.

In the beginning practise ten breath expulsions for one round, gradually increasing by ten expulsions each week until you reach a maximum of 120. Practise three rounds at each sitting. Alternatively you can practise 20 expulsions for each round, making six rounds (120 expulsions).

There are three breathing rates that you can use with *kapalabhati*:

- mild speed – one expulsion per second (60 per minute)
- medium speed – two expulsions per second (120 per minute)
- fast speed – four expulsions per second (240 per minute)

The beginner should practise the mild kapalabhati.

SURYA BHEDA PRANAYAMA

The Sanskrit word *surya* means sun and *bheda* means 'to pierce' to 'pass through'. *Surya bheda pranayama* activates the solar, right nostril (*pingala nadi*).

1 Sit in a meditative posture, preferably *padmasana* or *siddhasana*. Relax and close your eyes.
2 Raise your right hand and place your fingers in *vishnu mudra*. Close your left nostril with your third and fourth fingers. Inhale slowly,

deeply and quietly through your right nostril. Be totally aware as you inhale.
3 Close both nostrils and retain your breath. Apply the chin lock (*jalandhara bandha*) and the anal lock (*mulabandha*). Hold your breath without straining, for as long as is comfortable.
4 Release *mulabandha* first, then *jalandhara bandha*, and exhale slowly, deeply and quietly through your left nostril.

This completes one round. Without pausing, close your left nostril and again inhale through your right nostril, repeating steps 1–4.

Beginners should start with shorter breath retentions, gradually increasing the retention time as the lung capacity develops. You should also start with ten rounds, gradually increasing over a period of time to 40.

The *Gheranda Samhita* says that the practice of *surya bheda* destroys disease and death and awakens the *kundalini*. It awakens the *kundalini* by taking the *prana* into the *sushumna*. It purifies the brain and frontal sinuses. The digestion is stimulated and the nerves are invigorated and soothed – in fact the whole body is given a general tonic by this practice. It increases heat in the body so it is best to practise it during the winter months.

However, do not practise immediately before or after meals, because the energy is needed for digestion. Also do not practise late at night before going to sleep, because the *pingala nadi* will be activated, which will keep you awake.

Chandra Bheda Pranayama

Chandra means 'moon'. This *pranayama* is basically the same as the *surya bheda* except that all inhalations are through the left nostril, and the exhalations through the right.

In this practice the *prana* is channelled through the *ida* or *chandra nadi*, which cools the body system, whereas the *surya bheda* heats the system.

Note: Do not practise *surya bheda* and *chandra bheda* on the same day.

UJJAYI PRANAYAMA

The Sanskrit prefix *ud*, means 'to raise upwards', and *jaya* means 'the victorious'.

1 Sit in a comfortable meditative posture, close your eyes and relax.
2 With your mouth closed, slowly and smoothly inhale and exhale through both nostrils, partially closing the glottis in the throat. This produces an even and continuous hissing or soft snoring type of sound.
3 During the inhalation the air is felt on the soft roof palate, accompanied by the sibilant sound 'sa', due to the friction of the air. The exhalation is also felt on the soft roof palate and produces the aspirate sound 'ha'. During the inhalation (*puraka*) keep the abdominal muscles slightly contracted. Completely expand the lungs with air, by raising and expanding the ribs until the chest is thrust forward like a victorious warrior.
4 During the exhalation (*rechaka*) the abdominal muscles will naturally be more retracted. The duration of the exhalation is always longer than the inhalation, usually in the proportionate ratio of 1: 2. This means that if you inhale for five seconds, exhalation should be ten seconds.
5 Practise 5–20 rounds of *ujjayi pranayama*, starting with five and increasing by two rounds each week until you reach 20.

Advanced Ujjayi Pranayama

Advanced practitioners can perform *mulabandha* and *jalandhara bandha* with breath retention (*kumbhaka*).

1 After inhaling in *ujjayi*, completely close the glottis and perform *mulabandha* and *jalandhara bandha*.
2 After comfortably holding your breath (*kumbhaka*), first release *mulabandha*, then *jalandhara bandha*.
3 Exhale through your left nostril, by closing the right one with your thumb. This traditional way of exhalation through the left nostril requires less effort to breathe in the 1: 2 ratio. This is because

exhalation through one nostril will require double the time of inhalation through both nostrils, provided the force of breathing is constant.

Ujjayi pranayama can be practised at any time and in all positions – yoga postures, standing and walking – safely without breath retention. To balance the *prana* and *apana*, keep the length of the inhalation and exhalation the same, and breathe through both nostrils evenly.

This practice calms the mind and nervous system and is good for hypertension, anxiety and depression. It slows the heartbeat and reduces high blood pressure. It is also good for people suffering from insomnia, asthma, pulmonary diseases and heart diseases. It helps in regulating the blood pressure, endocrinal secretions and gastrointestinal activity, removes phlegm from the throat and cools the head.

It is also good for those people who do not cry (crying from positive emotions becomes purifying).

Ujjayi improves concentration when the awareness follows the breath, and helps to bring one to a meditative state by awakening one's psychic energies.

SITALI PRANAYAMA

Sitali (pronounced 'sheetali') is a cooling breath, it has a cooling and soothing effect on the body.

1. *Sitali* can be practised sitting in a meditative *asana* or standing.
2. Stick your tongue out just past the lips and curl or fold it lengthwise to form a tube. Inhale slowly and deeply through this tube, with a hissing sound, until your lungs are filled completely.
3. Withdraw your tongue, retain the breath and perform *jalandhara bandha*. Hold your breath for as long as is comfortable.
4. Release *jalandhara bandha* and slowly exhale through both nostrils.

This technique can be practised daily in the morning, beginning with ten rounds and gradually increasing to 40 rounds. It is best practised after *asana* and *pranayama* practice. Since it is a cooling breath, it should not be practised during the cold winter months.

Sitali cools the system and induces relaxation to the body and tranquillity to the mind. It purifies the blood, improves digestion and quenches thirst.

SITKARI PRANAYAMA

Sitkari (pronounced 'sheetkari') is also a cooling breath, and gives similar benefits to *sitali pranayama*.

Fold your tongue back so that the tip of the tongue touches the upper palate. Bring the teeth together, open the lips and inhale with a hissing sound through your teeth.

Differences Between *Sitali* and *Sitkari* Pranayamas

In *sitkari* the awareness is focused on the hissing sound.

In *sitali* the awareness is focused on the cooling sensation of the breath.

Sitkari can also be practised daily in the morning, beginning with ten rounds and gradually increasing to forty rounds.

BHRAMARI PRANAYAMA: HUMMING BEE BREATH

Bhramari improves the voice, making it become sweet and melodious. For this reason it is particularly good for vocal musicians or singers. It is also good for throat ailments, calms the mind and reduces blood pressure. It awakens the inner sound (*nada*).

1 Sit in a meditative *asana*, close your eyes and relax.
2 Inhale slowly and deeply through both nostrils.
3 Retain the breath and perform *jalandhara bandha*. Hold it for three to five seconds.
4 Release *jalandhara bandha* and raise your arms to close off all sound to your ears by placing your index fingers in them. Exhale through your nostrils with your mouth closed, making a high-pitched sound, like the humming of a bee, and feel this vibration in your brain.

Begin with five rounds and gradually increase to forty.

MURCHA PRANAYAMA

Murcha means 'to faint' or 'to expand'. This *pranayama* helps to expand the consciousness and induces relaxation and inner awareness.

You should not practise it if you suffer from heart disease, high blood pressure or vertigo.

1. Sit in *padmasana* or *siddhasana* with your hands on your knees, so that you are seated firmly and steady.
2. Inhale slowly and deeply, taking a complete yogic breath, then bend your head backwards and perform *shambhavi mudra* (see below) with your eyes open, concentrating at the point between the eyebrows.
3. Retain the breath for as long as is comfortable, and keep your arms straight, pressing your knees with your hands.
4. Exhale slowly as you relax your arms and close your eyes, bringing your head back to the upright position.
5. Relax and experience the calmness and tranquillity.

Variation: Retain the breath and perform *jalandhara bandha* instead of taking the head back and performing *shambhavi mudra*.

Shambhavi Mudra
(The Creative Power of Consciousness Mudra).

1. Sit in a meditative posture and with the eyes open gaze upward at the spiritual eye, the point between the eyebrows.
2. With the eyes held steadily, hold for as long as possible. When the eyes become tired, close them and relax them. Internalise your one-pointed awareness at the spiritual eye. After some practice you may see a light appear when the eyes are closed. Concentrate on that point of light, keeping it steadily held at the spiritual eye. Allow the mind and breath to become absorbed in contemplation.

Shambhari mudra can also be used in concentrating the mind internally in any *chakra*.

SAVITRI PRANAYAMA: THE RHYTHMIC BREATH

Savitri pranayama is a rhythmic, harmonizing breath, using a four-part breath ratio. The inhalation and exhalation are the same and the internal and external breath retentions are half that of the inhalation and exhalation.

The conventional ratio is 8: 4: 8: 4. This is the best rhythm to strengthen and rejuvenate the body, and it promotes optimum health. This rhythm is used as the basis of *pratyahara* (sense withdrawal) and *dharana* (concentration).

Different ratios of breath have different effects on the mind and body, as shown below.

- 4: 2: 4: 2.   Excellent for asthma, or convalescence from sickness or surgery. Good for a child beginning *pranayama*. This rhythm is good for a short duration, but if it is going to be practised over a long period, then one should try to extend the rhythm to 8: 4: 8: 4.
- 6: 3: 6: 3.   This is the best rhythm for controlling one's emotions, neurotic tendencies and manic depression. It harmonizes the emotional balance.
- 8: 4: 8: 4.   This rhythm strengthens and rejuvenates the body, promoting optimum health. It brings calmness to the body.
- 10: 5: 10: 5.   This increases the metabolism (speeds up the rate at which the body organs work). It is very beneficial for overcoming a sluggish circulation, laziness and procrastination.
- 12: 6: 12: 6.   This rhythm awakens the mind, gives alertness, retentive memory and clarity of thought and senses. It is good for spiritual development.
- 14: 7: 14: 7.   This calms the mind and senses, creating serenity of mind.
- 16: 8: 16: 8.   This is the Siddha Rhythm (the Master's Breath). It rejuvenates the body and promotes optimum health and longevity.

The technique for *savitri pranayama* is as follows.
1. Sit and relax in a meditative *asana* with your eyes closed.
2. Inhale slowly through both nostrils for a count of six seconds.
3. Retain the breath for three seconds.
4. Exhale slowly through both nostrils for six seconds.
5. Retain the breath externally for three seconds.

This completes one round. Practise nine rounds, then gradually increase to 27 as you progress. The duration of inhalation and exhalation can be increased gradually over a period of time, according to your strength and capacity, but do not force or strain it in any way.

SAVITRE PRANAYAMA

The difference between *savitre* and *savitri pranayama* is that the breathing ratio is reversed in *savitre*. The internal and external breath retentions are double the time of the inhalation and exhalation (1: 2: 1: 2). Beginners may start with the breathing ratio of 3: 6: 3: 6, gradually increasing to 27 rounds.

Over a period of time and according to your strength and capacity, increase the ratio to 6: 12: 6: 12, then 8: 16: 8: 16 maximum. Perform *jalandhara bandha* with the breath retentions. These rhythmic breathing ratios are named after the beautiful goddess Savitri, who governs the seasons of this planet. Savitri's consort is Savitu (Surya), god of the sun.

NAGA PRANAYAMA

This is a technique for purifying the skin. The breath is retained under pressure within the blood, which tries to release the carbon dioxide through the millions of pores in the skin. The skin discharges the carbon dioxide, increasing the temperature of the skin, which causes it to perspire, discharging its toxins.

This *pranayama* makes the skin softer and healthier. It is good for such skin conditions as psoriasis, eczema and acne. The benefits are more therapeutic than spiritual.

1. Sit in *vajrasana* with the eyes closed and the body relaxed.
2. Inhale slowly and deeply through both nostrils.
3. Retain the breath for a slow count of nine.
4. Still retaining the breath without letting any air escape, inhale and again retain the breath for another count of nine.
5. Repeat step once again. If your breathing capacity can still take more air into the lungs, then inhale and hold for a count of nine once more.
6. Exhale very slowly through both nostrils.
7. Practise two more rounds then lie down in total relaxation.

POLARITY BREATH (PRANIC BATH)

Each body cell has a polarity, magnetic in quality like the earth. When these cells are aligned and brought into balance then the psyche and body become balanced. The alignment of the cells is accomplished by drawing negative and positive currents of pranic energy through the body in a kind of cellular massage.

1. Lie on the floor in *shavasana* (relaxation pose) with your head pointing north and your feet pointing south. Close your eyes and relax.
2. Practise nine rounds of *savitri pranayama* (8: 4: 8: 4).
3. Now visualize the warmth and energy of the sun just over your head. Inhale this sun energy through the top of your head, gradually drawing it down to your feet, visualizing a warm golden *prana* flowing with the inhaling breath through your body. Allow the energy to filter out through the soles of your feet.
4. Retain the breath and visualize and feel a cool dynamic (moon) energy below your feet. Exhale from the feet up to the head, visualizing a cool silvery *prana* flowing through your body.
5. Practise 12 rounds slowly and rhythmically, until you experience a light, floating feeling. Then rest in deep relaxation.

Pranic Healing

All methods of healing are really indirect ways of awakening the life-energy (*prana*) within a dis-eased body. If the pranic currents in the body are unbalanced by unnatural living and improper breathing, the corresponding physiological processes are disturbed and thrown out of balance, causing various disorders and diseases.

Yogis who practise *pranayama* correctly regularly have access to a store of *prana*, which they are able to use for self-healing or for healing others. This pranic healing is imparted by concentration on and direction of the *prana* by the power of will to any part of the body.

Storing and Distributing *Prana*

1 Lie down on your back with the eyes closed, and completely relax. Place your left hand lightly over your solar plexus (just above the navel), and your right hand on top of it.
2 Breathe slowly and rhythmically. With each inhalation mentally direct the *prana* to the solar plexus. It also helps to visualize the *prana* entering and flowing through the body in the form of a healing blue or white light.
3 With each exhalation calmly and mentally direct and visualize this healing current of energy throughout the whole body. Distribute it to every bone, muscle, organ, nerve and cell.
4 Concentrate at the point between your eyebrows (spiritual eye) and affirm mentally, 'God's perfect light is perfectly present in all my body parts. Wherever that pranic healing light is manifest, there is perfection.'

Self-healing

1 Lie down with your eyes closed in *shavasana* (relaxation pose).
2 Visualize a ball of radiant white healing light just above the crown of your head.
3 Using the *savitri pranayama* ratio 8: 4: 8: 4, inhale to a count of eight seconds through both nostrils. Simultaneously visualize and feel

that you are drawing in a stream of pure white healing light through the soles of your feet up to your head, energizing and revitalizing your whole body and the chakras as it flows through you.
4   Hold your breath for a count of four seconds.
5   Exhale to a count of eight seconds, visualizing a stream of pure white light flowing down from your head to your feet, cleansing all the toxins and impurities from your body out through the soles of your feet.
6   Retain the breath out for a count of four seconds.
7   Practise five more rounds.
8   Return to normal breathing, but breathe with long, slow, deep rhythmic breaths.
9   Inhale and visualize healing pranic energy flowing from the soles of your feet up the back of your body to your head.
10 Exhale from your face down the front of your body to your feet.
11 Circulate the *prana* from back to front three times.
12 Now, visualize the *prana* flowing up the front of your body as you inhale, and flowing down the back as you exhale, three times.
13 Inhale and visualize the *prana* flowing from left to right three times.
14 Exhale and visualize the pranic energy flowing from right to left three times.
15 Relax completely and concentrate on the spiritual eye. Affirm mentally, 'God's perfect health and pranic energy pervades my body cells. This body is well. God's healing light is shining brightly in every cell.'

6

PRATYAHARA

In the preceding chapters we have studied four of the eight limbs of Patanjali's yoga. Let us briefly review them.

The practice of *yama* and *niyama* helps to remove restlessness, desires, delusions and wrong attachments from the mind due to misunderstanding and ignorance.

The practice of *asana* trains us to make the body steady with ease and comfort, in order to ensure that the mind becomes still and quiet in preparation for meditation.

The practice of *pranayama* purifies and removes distractions from the mind.

Now we come to the fifth limb, *pratyahara*. This is covered in only two sutras.

> Pratyahara *is the interiorization of the mind, by reversing the senses' outward attention from external objects to their source within (the divine Self).*
>
> The Yoga Sutras of Patanjali 2:54

> *By conscious interiorization of the mind, the senses function intelligently and in harmony without ego-mind interference. One acquires complete mastery over all the senses.*
>
> 2:55

The practices of *yama, niyama, asana, pranayama* and *pratyahara* are concerned with the body and brain. They constitute the outer phase of yoga. The final three limbs, *dharana, dhyana* and *samadhi* constitute the inner phase of yoga, and are concerned with the reconditioning of mind.

Pratyahara is a state in which the attention does not externalize itself. Usually as you look at something, listen to some sound, smell or touch something, your attention is drawn out of yourself. In *pratyahara* the attention is directed inwards.

Through the practice of *asana* and *pranayama* one turns the mind's attention within, being totally aware of where the impulse to breathe in and breathe out arises. Total attention and awareness of that is itself *pratyahara*, or drawing one's attention into and within oneself.

The Senses

The five components of creation – ether, air, fire water and earth – have given us our five senses: hearing, feeling, sight, taste and smell respectively.

The soul (the true Self) shines by its own light; it is the true source of intelligence which gives life to the body, mind and senses. Without the life-force of the soul, the body, mind and senses cannot function at all.

Primarily (as young children prove) the senses are the first instruments to gather knowledge or perception from the world. The reason I use the expression 'to gather' is because awareness of sense-perceptions arises only if the information delivered by the senses reaches the mind. Without mind there is no recorded perception and so the senses become useless as instruments.

When the mind receives the collected information from the senses it examines, analyses and discriminates what it has received and acts upon it.

But what makes the senses go out and gather information? It is curiosity. So curiosity has to exist in the mind to determine it to send the senses out to gather information to satisfy that curiosity. But the more you try to satisfy your mind's curiosity, the more curiosity is generated, because each piece of information triggers more questions.

The mind has this inborn curiosity because it is looking for meaning. It wants to enlarge the whole informational picture until it makes sense. So curiosity, or the desire to find out and know things, is a search for meaning.

So why does the attempt of the mind and senses to find meaning in life fail so often? The senses are the means for gathering experience. Experience may be divided into pleasant and unpleasant, like and dislike. Each sensory experience leaves an impression on the mind. For example, when you first perceive an apple and touch it, smell it and taste it, you have knowledge of an apple. An impression (*samskara*) is immediately formed in the subconscious mind, and at any time this *samskara* can generate a memory of the object – the apple and knowledge of the apple.

After accumulating a number of experiences that are alike, the mind forms an idea about them. So now the ego, the 'I' which is born of ignorance, which *is* ignorance, intervenes, disregarding the truth or the reality that all these experiences come and go.

The ego says: 'That was beautiful, I want to keep it. This is horrible, I want to avoid it.' But neither of these is possible. If the beautiful thing we saw is not present, the mind which registered the experience as memory goes on wanting it; and what is even more unfortunate, the mind also remembers an unpleasant experience and goes on fearing it. It is not there, but you know it might come again. It also might not, again, but the mind retains the impression of that momentary experience of pleasure or of displeasure, and out of these are born desire and dislike. When the momentary experience of pleasure born of sense-contact is allowed to leave an impression on the mind, the mind becomes coloured by it, so that afterwards wherever you look, that thing goes on in the mind – 'I want that, I must have it', or 'I desire something, but I fear it may not happen.'

Gradually the obstinate efforts to repeat pleasurable experiences and avoid unpleasant ones lead one to abandon the initial search – the search for meaning. Instead one becomes addicted to pleasure and comfort, not understanding that pleasure is not in the objects but in the condition of the mind, and that happiness is not in the objects but within one's own Self. Our lives become governed by desire and attachment, and the so-called need to defend what we think we have.

The other intervening phenomenon is a dulling of the senses due to over-repetition. The drug addict starts with marijuana and goes on to taking stronger drugs like cocaine and heroin. The smoker smokes more cigarettes. The drinker drinks more, and ends up becoming an alcoholic. The relationship that becomes more and more sexual, without love (based on physical self-gratification) soon becomes dull and boring, and so one or both partners continually look to more stimulating and degrading sexual practices, where the partners are mere objects of stimulation. Whether it is drugs, alcohol, sex, smoking, coffee or sugar, indulgence in any pleasure dulls the sensitivity of the senses and the nervous system. In the end it will either bore you or enslave you, and in that there is no freedom, beauty or joy. The initial stimulus is no longer strong enough to cause pleasure. The initial sharpness and awareness of the sense-experience wears off and the senses need a stronger one in order for the ego to have the kind of pleasure it expects.

The way the ego relates to experience is also wrong, in that it wants to possess the objects of its attachment. The ego is frustrated by the fleetingness of pleasure and wants to eternalize it through possession. In fact, possession is a delusion. We do not even own what we eat. We just recycle energies, and not even that process is a conscious one. Possessiveness 'freezes' the relationship with the object or person.

Instead of using our senses to discover the meaning at the interface of any process of relating, we want to 'have' this or that experience out of it. What gets lost again is the meaning, the teaching that we receive. We unwittingly refer to the *ego* rather than the *Self*.

Please understand that it is not the object that binds or enslaves you. It is the *identification* of the thought with the object that causes desire, possessiveness, attachment and fear. It is the identification and labelling of things as 'desirable' and 'undesirable' by the ego that causes all the problems. The mind labels a sensation or experience desirable, which automatically makes its opposite or absence undesirable – pleasure creates pain. The sensation becomes a feeling at the point when thought arises to label the sensations. The labelling creates a division between the thought and the experience. In pure experiencing there is no labelling. In the state of pure awareness, the mind is undivided and steady. If the mind seeks the experience of something other than the inner joy and inner peace of the self, the awareness of its own nature is lost. That is why self-discipline is emphasized by the yoga Masters, not as something important in itself, but as a condition in which the subject becomes aware of itself.

When the futility of desire and the pursuit of sensory objects is seen, the mind is left with the feeling that something is lacking. That which is lacking is soul-fulfilment, inner joy and inner peace. It is forgetfulness of our true blissful self. Due to the soul's forgetfulness of its own blissful nature, it tries to satisfy itself with the illusory and fleeting joys of sensory pleasures. In all of us, the soul is inwardly conscious of losing its blissful contact with God, the source of all joy, peace and love, and can never remain satisfied with the limited pleasures of the senses.

> The true purpose of life is to know God. Worldly temptations were given to help you develop discrimination: will you prefer sense pleasures, or will you choose God? Pleasures seem alluring at first, but if you choose them, sooner or later you will find yourself enmeshed in endless troubles and difficulties.
>
> Loss of health, of peace of mind, and of happiness is the lot of everyone who succumbs to the lure of sense pleasures. Infinite joy, on the other hand, is yours once you know God.
>
> Every human being will have, eventually, to learn this great lesson of life!
>
> Paramhansa Yogananda, from *The Essence of Self-Realization* by Sri Kriyananda

MASTERY OF THE SENSES

Lord Krishna warns us in the *Bhagavad Gita* that if the senses are not controlled, the mind will be distracted and captivated by attachment to sensory experiences, leading to forgetfulness of one's true Self-nature.

> Just as a tortoise draws in its limbs within its shell, the wise yogi, fixed in higher consciousness, disconnects the senses from their objects of perception at will, resulting in steadiness of mind.
>
> Those who deprive the senses from experiencing their objects experience that they still crave for them. These sense cravings only come to an end when one attains a higher knowledge and realizes the Self.
>
> The force of the stimulated senses is sufficient to disturb even the most discriminating of aspirants in the midst of all their efforts for self-control.
>
> Having brought the senses under control one should be joined in yoga with the mind ever established in Me. The wisdom of one who has mastered the senses becomes steadfast and unwavering.
>
> The senses become attached to an object when it is continually thought of. As a result of such involvement, the desire to enjoy the object arises. When such a desire is unfulfilled or obstructed, anger arises.

Anger clouds discrimination and one becomes easily illusioned, losing the memory of one's own true self. From loss of memory one loses the faculty of discrimination and eventually from the confusion of intelligence misses the goal of human life – Self- realization.

However those who can supervise the involvement between the senses and sense-objects by exercising enlightened self-control, and who become free from craving and false repression, attain inner calmness and peace.

In that inner calmness and inner joy comes the end of all sorrows. For the intelligence of the calm-minded soon becomes firmly established in the Self.

For one whose mind and senses are unsteady, there is no knowledge of the Self. When the mind is restless it cannot concentrate or meditate; it has no peace. Without inner peace, how can there be joy?

Just as a boat on the sea is carried away by the wind in a storm, so can a person's intelligence and understanding be carried away by the force of sense desire.

Therefore, one whose senses are completely mastered, becomes firmly established in wisdom of the Self.

Just as the vast ocean remains calm and unperturbed, even though many rivers flow into it from all sides, so a person should remain undisturbed by the continued arising of sense-desires. One who is controlled by desire cannot attain true peace.

True inner peace arises when all sense-desires are transcended and orientated to higher levels of consciousness; and when one acts free from identification with the false ego, and the illusion of the sense of 'I' and 'mine'.

Bhagavad Gita 2:58–71

THE PRACTICE OF *PRATYAHARA*

The difference between a Master of yoga and an ordinary worldly person is that the yogi experiences true joy and inner peace by inwardly reversing the searchlight of perception from the senses to the divine source within, *consciously at will*. The worldly person, whose ego-mind identifies with and is attached to the senses, becomes disunited from the inner source of joy and peace – the Self. Instead, the worldly person suffers restlessly with anger, fear and loss of inner peace and joy.

The worldly person can only disconnect the mind from the senses in the *subconscious* state of ordinary sleep. In the deep inertia of sleep, the life-force that connects the mind with the senses reverts back to the

Self-conscious force of the soul. In this state of sleep there is no consciousness of 'I'. There is no desire to experience, there is no ego-sense. In sleep you are not aware that 'I am', otherwise you are awake! What remains is pure experiencing – there is no contact with the objects of the senses, and since there is no contact, the mind is not divided. That is why you do not experience pain or suffering at all during sleep.

In the dream state during sleep, the senses of perception are still and absorbed in the mind. It is only the mind that is actively operating during dream; it becomes both the subject and the object. During the wakeful state objects exist independently of the mind. Whether you are asleep or awake the objects are always there. However, in dreams the objects exist only as long as there is the mind to create them and for as long as the dream lasts. When you awake from your sleep all the dream objects disappear.

Yoga Nidra: The Psychic Sleep of the Yogis

Yoga nidra is one of the best techniques for developing awareness and to achieve a state of *pratyahara*.

Yoga psychology realizes that relaxation is a natural behaviour and can be relearned by those whose faulty living and thinking habits have caused unnatural, neurotic, over-reactive behaviour. Yoga techniques develop the faculty of concentration as well as bringing about relaxation. Concentration, the ability to focus the mind on one thought form, is a very effective way of removing the mind from worrying and anxiety-provoking thoughts. *Yoga nidra* is therefore not only a powerful form of relaxation, but its repeated practice aids in the development of the mental faculties as well. Since relaxation is the first step in the development of meditation, *yoga nidra* is the ideal first practice of *pratyahara* for the student of yoga.

In the *yoga nidra* state one is completely and totally relaxed on all levels – physical, mental and emotional. In this state the brainwave pattern changes and becomes slower, from the usual busy, waking beta level to the deeper, slower alpha level.

In *yoga nidra* one does not actually sleep in an unconscious way. The body, brain and nervous system are completely relaxed, while the consciousness remains totally alert, awake and aware. In this state of consciousness, which is on the borderline between sleep and wakefulness, there is contact with the subconscious and unconscious mind – the deeper layers of your personality. Through the practice of *yoga nidra* we are able to recognize, release and eliminate our suppressions, fears, phobias, neuroses and deep-rooted tensions – all things that condition our conscious thoughts and experiences in a negative way.

The main elements of *yoga nidra* practice are:

1 **Body relaxation/awareness and rotation of consciousness**: The consciousness is rotated through the different parts of the body a number of times to reduce the mind's attention on external stimuli, thus introverting the mind, and relaxing the physical body.
2 *Pratyahara*: The mind is very rebellious; it does the opposite of what you want it to do. So in *yoga nidra* we deliberately focus our attention on external things with complete awareness. In this way the mind loses interest in the external things and naturally withdraws and goes within.
3 **Breath awareness**: With breath awareness, there is no attempt to force or change the breath. You just silently watch the natural breath flow in and out. This practice takes you into a deeper state of physical relaxation.
4 **Awareness of feelings or emotions**: Through the practice of visualization, using stories and images, we are able to awaken or recall, and voluntarily bring to the surface, suppressed and deep-rooted feelings and emotions from the subconscious and unconscious levels of our minds. When these deep-rooted fears and anxieties rise to the surface, we watch them with awareness and detachment – we recognize them, then release them. This process can be useful to cleanse unwanted patterns from the mental field and emotional life.
5 **Affirmation**: Having released the negative feelings and impressions from the subconscious it is important to implant a positive affirmation. During the deep relaxation of *yoga nidra*, the deeper layers of the subconscious are very impressionable to suggestions from the conscious will. Affirm with conviction, faith and deep concentration the statement of truth which you aspire to absorb into your life.

Practise *yoga nidra* in *shavasana* (the relaxation pose), in a quiet, warm room. Wear loose, comfortable clothing and lie down on a folded blanket or rug. Keep the body warm by covering yourself with a blanket. Once *yoga nidra* has begun, there must be no physical movement. One must remain completely aware and awake throughout the whole process.

You can either be guided through the process by a teacher who instructs clearly and slowly in a relaxed tone of voice, or be guided by listening to a *yoga nidra* cassette tape especially recorded for this purpose.

OTHER *PRATYAHARA* PRACTICES

- First practise a few rounds of *kapalabhati* (see chapter 4) and *bhastrika pranayama* (see chapter 5), then practise *yoni mudra* (see chapter 4).
- Practise *savitri pranayama* (see chapter 5) in the ratio 8: 4: 8: 4. This breathing ratio is used for the basis of *pratyahara* and concentration.
- Practise the *sarvangasana* (shoulder stand) (see chapter 2), followed by *halasana* (plough pose), then practise *karnapidasana* (ear-knee pose) (see below). It is by relaxing for some time in *karnapidasana* that you can experience *pratyahara*.
- Practise *japa*, (the repetition of a mantra or a Name of God – see chapter 3).
- Practise *nada* (listening to inner sounds – see chapter 3).
- Practise *kirtan* (chanting devotionally – see chapter 3), first loudly, then softly, whispered, mentally and superconsciously.
- Practise Kriya Yoga (see chapter 8).

Halasana (plough pose) and *karnapidasana* (knee-ear pose)

Method:
The plough is practised after the shoulder stand (*sarvangasana*).

1. From the shoulder stand exhale and lower your legs gradually to the floor behind your head.
2. If you can bring your toes to the floor without any back strain then

stretch out your arms away from your back, and clasp your hands together to give a good stretch. Then stretch your hands behind your head to touch your toes. Relax in this pose, breathing normally.
3 If you are supple enough you can exhale as you bend both knees and drop them down to the floor, either side of the ears. This is called *karnapidasana* (knee-ear pose)
4 Wrap your arms around your knees with your hands clasped together. Relax, breathe normally.
5 To come out of the pose, stretch your arms on the floor palms down away from your back. Press against the floor with your arms and palms so that you can gradually lower your back to the floor with control. Completely relax and breathe normally.

Caution: Do not practise *halasana* or *karnapidasana* if you suffer from:

- sciatica
- high blood pressure
- detached retina

Females are advised not to practise during menstruation.

Benefits:
- The plough (*halasana*) stretches the entire spine, particularly the cervical area.
- It tones and stretches the posterior muscles of the entire body.
- It stimulates the nerves and tones the internal organs and glands, especially the kidneys, liver and pancreas.
- It regulates the thyroid gland in the throat.
- It strengthens the heart and improves blood circulation.

The benefits here apply to *karnapidasana* as well.

7

DHARANA

Once the senses are mastered through *pratyahara*, they can be restored to serve the realization of the Self, instead of being misguided in serving the ignorance projected by the ego. Then the mind is ready for the next stage – interiorization of the mind. Calmly focusing the full attention of the mind and consciousness on one point to the exclusion of everything else – this is *dharana* (concentration). *Dharana* comes from the word *dhri*, 'to hold firm'.

In *The Yoga Sutras of Patanjali*, *dharana* is simply described in one sutra:

> Concentration is the binding of the mind's attention (focused awareness) to one particular point (to the exclusion of everything else).
>
> *Yoga Sutras* 3:1

Patanjali is not referring to concentration as generalized attention, where the mind is still engaged in thought-processes, but to the yoga technique of 'one-pointed' (*ekagrata*) concentration: a continuous flow of consciousness inwards, either on an internal object (*antara-visaya*), or an externalized object (*bahya-visaya*). The internal objects refer to points within the body – the navel, the heart, the point between the eyebrows, particularly the higher *chakras*. The external object is an idea or image of an object that the mind's attention is calmly focused on from within.

What is attention? It is the focusing of awareness upon a single object or idea to the exclusion of all else. Simple attention to our *lack* of awareness is the awakening of awareness.

Our concentration can either be focused or diffused. If you focus the scattered rays of sunlight into a single beam through a magnifying glass, they can burn a piece of paper, whereas the diffused rays cannot do this. Similarly, the mind's mental rays are usually dissipated on various objects and thoughts, but if they are collected and brought into sharp focus and clarity as a powerful single beam of concentration, one can burn away all the impurities (*samskaras*) of the mind.

Concentration is necessary in all actions if we are to achieve anything successfully and safely. You can understand the importance of safety if you imagine what could happen if you were driving your car along a busy road with your attention scattered on other things, or if you imagine your dentist drilling your teeth with his head turned talking to his assistant nurse.

Even in the simple actions of everyday living, our concentration and awareness is lacking. We forget that the bread is toasting on the grill and find it is on fire! We awake in the morning to find that we left the tap or the electric lights on all night.

The difficulty in understanding the term 'concentration' in the yogic sense is that commonly, concentration is associated with effort and tenseness. One concentrates in order to defend, possess or achieve something. In this sense, concentration is ego-motivated; it is an outward effort of the will, charged with the energy of the feelings, instead of a steady effortless flow of will-power. So in concentration the less effort the better! That is also the reason why Patanjali suggests that *pranayama* qualifies the mind for concentration. In *pranayama* we already have a glimpse of something beyond the self, and so when it comes to concentration there is virtually no effort, especially when it is done after practising *pranayama*. Sri Kriyananda writes in his *14 Steps to Joy*:

> *When the will, instead of being focussed on doing or accomplishing anything, is united inwardly to the purified intellect in a simple act of becoming, divine enlightenment ensues.*

ACHIEVING DHARANA

How do we have to change our approach to achieve *dharana*?

- Relax the mind and body. The less tension there is in the mind and body, the easier it is for the mind to focus its attention. Relaxing the body in the correct posture is necessary for concentration because it allows the energies in the spine to flow upward to the higher brain centres without obstruction. Relaxation – the gate to openness and receptivity – helps to counteract the contractive force of the self-limited ego-sense.
- Steady the mind and body. A steady pose gives concentration of mind. The practice of yoga *asanas* will enable you to regain steadiness of the body and mind, so that without distraction, the attention may be focused upon the object of concentration.
- Calm the breathing. If you pay attention to your breathing, you will come to know the degree of distractedness of the mind. The less distracted it is, the calmer the breath. The practice of *pranayama* (see chapter 5) brings calmness and equilibrium to the mind, enabling it to concentrate without distraction.
- Cultivate willingness. Remember that *dharana* has nothing to do with achieving a mundane goal, so there is no practical immediacy, there is no deadline, no effort. There is a *willingness* rather than an ego-motivated *will* that starts operating.
- Cultivate interest and attention. Concentration also requires interest and attention. We have to create interest to induce attention, because the mind finds it difficult to focus on an uninteresting object but easy to focus on an attractive one.

How do we know when the mind is concentrated? It happens when there is no sense of time. When we are deep in concentration, time passes by unnoticed. If we are reading a book and are interested in it, we give it all our attention, to the extent of not noticing the time at all. It is only when we stop reading and put the book down that we are surprised to find that a few hours have passed unnoticed. The mind is concentrated when one's interest and attention are sharply focused on a limited area (without the interference of thoughts) in the present moment – not the past nor the future, but *now*.

It is stated in the yogic scripture the *Kurma Purana* that if the mind is focused on something for 12 seconds, it is *dharana*. Twelve *dharanas* make a *dhyana* (meditation) and twelve *dhyanas* will be a *samadhi* (superconsciousness).

The Boy Who Concentrated on a Buffalo

There is a story that is often told to yoga students by swamis to demonstrate the aim of concentration and meditation.

One day a boy was inspired by the peace radiating from a holy man and asked to learn meditation from him. The guru taught him to meditate on a deity, but after some time had passed, the guru noticed that his disciple was not making progress in meditation, so he asked the boy what interested him most. The boy immediately told him that his buffalo was closest to his mind and heart. With this knowledge, the guru told the boy to go and sit in the meditation room and concentrate with complete attention on the buffalo.

The next day the guru knocked at the door of the meditation room and asked the boy to come out. For a few moments there was no reply, only silence. After a short while the boy replied in a deep voice, 'I'm sorry master but I cannot leave the room, as the door is too narrow for my large horns to go through!'

The guru then realized that the boy had achieved such deep concentration and meditation that it had caused him to enter *samadhi* (superconsciousness), in which he had lost his individuality and had become one with the buffalo.

It is not a real loss of one's nature but it is as if one's personality has been completely taken over by the object of meditation. For the time being the boy really thought that he was the buffalo he had concentrated on. Therefore it is suggested that one concentrates and meditates upon something that inspires and uplifts the consciousness, so as to grow into the likeness of that image. The moral of this story is that deep concentration on something that interests us and that we love unites us with it.

Fixing Your Mind on God

We all have the ability to concentrate on something that interests us, whether it is painting a picture, reading a book, driving a car or cooking a meal. But there are very few people who can concentrate or fix their minds on God or the Self within. During the 24 hours of the day the rays of the mind are mostly scattered in every direction except that of God. How much time do we actually give to concentrating on God? If you kept a diary of how much time your attention was on God, you may be surprised that out of 24 hours, it could be less than five minutes! Are we really that busy that we cannot think of God? What stops us from giving more attention to the divine? Is it lack of faith or interest? Throughout the day the mind cannot see anything beyond self-interest (ego-sense); its identification and attention is mostly with the sense of ego ('I am this body-mind-personality complex'). The mind concentrates on acquiring wealth, fame, power and indulging in worldly pleasures to the exclusion of the most important aim in life, Self-realization, to realize the true source of your life – God. God, the Supreme Reality who is truth, ever-existing, ever-conscious and ever-new bliss, who is without cause and is the cause of all causes, is the source of us. God is our true security, in the divine, we live, move and have our being. To live without the conscious awareness and presence of God is to live a limited life in which the mind seeks for pleasure, but finds pain and suffering.

If our consciousness is not attuned to the presence of God within us, if we are not centred in the conscious awareness of God, but are identified with the mind, which is limited to time, space and causation, then we do not experience that true lasting inner peace, harmony, divine love and inner joy or bliss that we are all seeking.

The individual soul-consciousness, which we are, contains all the qualities of the divine – love, peace, joy, light, wisdom – and we have have only to find out, know and realize it.

Our true purpose in life is to take up the one idea of awakening to our divine nature within and remaining in that conscious awareness and presence of the reality of God.

Take up one idea. Make that one idea your life; think of it; dream of it; live on that idea. Let the brain, muscles, nerves, every part of your body be full of that idea, and just leave every other idea alone. This is the way to success, and this is the way great spiritual giants are produced!

Swami Vivekananda, from *Teachings of Swami Vivekananda*

The Practice of Concentration

To enter deep concentration:

1 Relax your body and maintain a firm and steady *asana*.
2 Relax your mind, calm your breath and control your life-force with *pranayama* (see chapter 5).
3 Still your senses by reverting them back, inwardly, to their source through *pratyahara* (see chapter 6).
4 With your thoughts diminished, collect the rays of your mind and calmly focus them with interest and attention on one point of concentration. This is *dharana*.

Meditation begins when all the mental energies of the mind are focused on one idea alone. It is when the mind is concentrated inwardly on the presence of God in the soul.

In deep, 'one-pointed' concentration there is no consciousness of the body, time or surroundings. There is an increase of energy which magnetizes the spine and progressively rises to the higher chakras, taking one into an expansive state of consciousness, in which one can realize the omnipresence of God.

Interiorizing and Concentrating the Mind

Awareness of the Breath

To overcome mental restlessness, sit in a comfortable meditative posture and concentrate with focused attention inwardly on your natural breath. Make no attempts to control your breath in any way; simply observe its natural inward and outward flow, as if you were watching the tide flow in and out on the beach. Do not allow your mind to wander; if it does then gently bring it back to the awareness of the breath.

Concentration on the Spiritual Eye

Continue to observe the natural flow of the breath attentively. When it is calm, focus your concentration on the point between the eyebrows (the spiritual eye). Concentration on this point acts like a magnet, drawing the pranic energy flow upwards, interiorizing the energy in the higher brain centres.

Concentration on a Mantra

Sound vibration is the most powerful force in changing the mind; it is very easy for the mind to concentrate on. When the mind is absorbed in the transcendental sound of a mantra, it rises into a blissful state of superconsciousness. *Mantra* means 'that which protects or frees the mind'. Mantra protects and liberates the mind from restless thoughts and negativity; it transforms the energy of the mind to a higher level of consciousness. Each syllable of a mantra is empowered with divine spiritual power. When the mantra is repeated with concentration and meaning, it vibrates in the mind to produce harmony and balance. It also activates the chakras.

Of all mantras, *om* is the nearest symbol of God for helping the concentration of the mind (see chapter 3).

Hong Sau

A very good mantra for increasing concentration, calming the mind and one's consciousness of peace is the two-syllabled mantra *hong sau* (pronounced 'hong saw'), which is the inner sound of the inhaling and exhaling breath. It corresponds to the pranic currents in the spine, in the *ida* and the *pingala nadis*. When the breath is coming in there is a rising of energy in the spine that corresponds to a mental attitude of going outward. When the breath is going out there is a downward movement in the spine that corresponds to an inwardness of the energy in the body and consciousness.

Hong sau means 'I am He'. It is the affirmation of the self, affirming the self, offering to the divine.

When the breath flows in we mentally follow it with the chant *hong* and when the breath flows out we mentally follow it with the chant *sau*. Sri Kriyananda says:

> *When the breath is coming in, in a sense we are affirming 'I', but in that dissolving sense that prepares us to offer it back into the Infinite. When we say* sau *and then come back into the consciousness of 'I' again, with the incoming breath, we are affirming the opposite, 'He is I', and therefore this 'I' is more transcendent and not just this ego. Each helps the other.*

In fact this is also a mantra that you find used in India, called *soham*. (*Hong Sau* reversed becomes *soham*.)

To prepare for the practice of *hong sau*, follow this procedure.

1 Sit upright in a comfortable meditation posture, close the eyes and relax completely. To relax your body completely, inhale with a deep breath and tense your whole body. Exhale and relax. Practise tensing and relaxing three times, then completely relax and *feel* the relaxation.
2 Now continue to remain relaxed as you practise six to nine rounds of *loma pranayama* (see chapter 5). This is a three-part equal-breath ratio, breathing through both nostrils. Inhale for a count of 12, hold the breath for a count of 12, exhale for 12 (12: 12: 12). If this is not within your lung capacity, halve it to 6: 6: 6.
3 Remain still and concentrate your relaxed attention at the point between the eyebrows. Let go of all thoughts and be totally centred in the present moment – here and now. Keep your attentive awareness on the natural breath as you continue to look into the spiritual eye. If your mind wanders, gently bring it back to the practice of watching the breath with awareness. Interiorize your mind by deepening the concentration until you become completely absorbed.

Now move on to the practice itself.

1 Before you begin, exhale deeply, then when the breath naturally begins to flow in, mentally follow it with the sound *hong*.
2 When the breath naturally flows out, mentally follow it with the sound *sau*.

3 With the attention flowing to the spiritual eye (the point between the eyebrows) and concentrating on the breath (not the breathing process, but the air that enters the nostrils), feel it entering the nostrils, then feel it entering and awakening the spiritual eye in the frontal lobe of the brain.
4 Continue looking inwardly into the spiritual eye as you concentrate on the breath, mentally following the inhalation with *hong* and the exhalation with *sau* until your mind has become focused and still, lengthening and enjoying the pauses or spaces between the natural breaths.

This deep concentration practice gives the enjoyment of deep inner peace, so practise it with the feeling of peace, not as a mechanical exercise. Enjoy the peace, particularly between the breaths.

OTHER TECHNIQUES THAT HELP CONCENTRATION

TRATAK (STEADY GAZING) AND VISUALIZATION

This technique was covered in chapter 4. The gaze is directed without blinking and with complete concentration on an external object, such as a candle flame, the moon, a bright star, a mandala, a beautiful flower, or the eyes of a picture of your guru or a saint.

To practise *tratak* on a picture of your guru, Jesus Christ, Krishna or a saint, sit in a comfortable and relaxed posture and place the picture of your choice in front of you at eye level, and at a distance of one arm's length. With the eyes open gaze steadily at it with full attention and interest, then close your eyes after a minute or two and visualize the face and eyes of the Master, guru or saint you have been gazing at. Attune yourself to the consciousness of these Masters by visualizing them at the spiritual eye. Feel their presence, love, joy, light and energy within the lotus of your heart.

Remember, also, that no matter how much love you direct towards the personalized image (saint, guru, deity, etc) the object of devotional concentration should always be regarded as just one expression of God, otherwise we cease to feel the unity behind the multiplicity of manifestations – the unmanifested godhead, that which is not limited to time or space, that which is omnipresent, omnipotent and omniscient. We need to go beyond personality worship and worship of the form and attune ourselves to the divine Consciousness that gives and expresses love, light, joy and wisdom through the form of personality.

JAPA

Japa is the repetition of any of the Names of God for developing devotion and concentrating the mind on God, and is described in chapter 3. The repetition may be either aloud, whispered or silently to oneself. *Japa* is usually practised with the use of *mala* beads or a rosary, containing 108 beads. The significance of the number 108 is that the ancient yogis worked out that the normal person breathes 21,600 breaths in 24 hours; 200 times 108 equals 21,600. One hundred and eight is also divisible by nine, which is a spiritual number.

Mental *japa*, when repeated with concentration and an attitude of total surrender to God, prepares the mind for deep meditation. The constant practice of *japa* purifies the mind and reverses the thought-current from external objects, inwardly towards God.

To practise *japa*, sit in a comfortable meditation posture and concentrate either on the heart chakra (*anahata*) or on the space between the eyebrows (the spiritual eye) – see page 86. By fixing the concentration of the mind and closed eyes on the inner spiritual eye, the mind is easily controlled.

Hold your *japa mala* or rosary in your right hand. Starting with the first small bead next to the larger *sumeru* bead, hold it between your right thumb and middle finger and with concentration repeat your mantra once. Now move on to the next small bead and repeat the mantra. Continue in this way around the *mala* with each bead until you have complete 108 mantras. When you arrive back at the *sumeru* bead you should not cross over it to start the next round, but turn the *mala* and begin from the last bead before the *sumeru*.

KIRTAN

Kirtan or chanting, which is also discussed in chapter 3, is an excellent way of directing and focusing the energies of the mind inward towards God. Devotional chanting awakens the natural love and devotion in the heart. It can inspire us to want to know and be closer to God. It gives us the taste of bliss that is the Self. Chanting also invokes an atmosphere of love, joy and peace.

Before you begin to chant ask yourself, 'Who am I chanting to and why?' This is important if you are to transcend the ego-sense. When we chant, we should feel that the Lord is seated within our heart. Chant with love and devotion and absorb the mind in God alone. As you chant, listen attentively to the words and feel the energy and vibrational power of the chants. Keep your eyes closed and concentrate either on the spiritual eye (*ajna chakra*) or the heart chakra.

Begin the chant aloud, filling the body and mind with the words and rhythms of the chanting, then gradually decrease the volume while increasing the inner experience of the chant until, at the superconscious stage, you turn internal vibrations into spiritual realizations. Paramhansa Yogananda used to say to his disciples that 'chanting is half the battle'. These inspiring words from a great Master are very encouraging for anyone who is truly seeking God.

8

DHYANA

Dharana (concentration) is the first stage of meditation. The second stage is *dhyana*, unbroken concentration or absorption.

> *Meditation is the continuous and effortless flow of attentive awareness towards the object of concentration.*
>
> The Yoga Sutras of Patanjali 3:2

There is a difference between concentration and meditation. In concentration (*dharana*), the attention is focused on a small, limited area (the object of concentration). If at that time only one thought or idea functions in the mind, that is meditation (*dhyana*). In meditation there is not even a suggestion of distraction. If there is awareness of distraction, you are only concentrating and not meditating.

The difference between concentration and meditation is that in concentration there is a peripheral awareness and distraction, whereas in meditation the attention is not disturbed, there are no distractions at all. In meditation the mind becomes one with its object, it is only conscious of itself and the object.

WHY WE NEED TO MEDITATE

People approach meditation for many different reasons, the most obvious being for release of stress, peace of mind, relaxation, an increase in energy and healing. Some people meditate in an attempt to solve their problems; they sit to think or to explore the mind. Others may even meditate to escape from life and reality, or to experience a 'high', like some drug-induced experience. For many people meditation is difficult to understand and many give up after their first few attempts, but nothing comes easily in life. First we need to have a sincere aspiration to realize the Self and know God. Secondly, we need to persevere with our practice by making a conscious effort until we succeed in experiencing the fruits of deep meditation – inner peace, inner joy, divine energy and deep calmness.

Meditation certainly contributes to our physical, mental and emotional well-being, but the true aim is to go beyond the limits of the finite mind and free ourselves from its thought waves (*vrittis*). In other words, it involves quietening the movements of the mind, bringing it to a state of undisturbed silence, to realize and express that pure consciousness which is the reflection of God within us. When the thought waves are brought under control, and the mind becomes quiet, then we are able to experience the higher states of consciousness, in which the light of consciousness, turned in upon itself, can experience divine union with God. In this elevated state of consciousness one transcends the mind, intellect and ego-sense to experience the true nature of the Self, which is *Sat-Chit-Ananda* (ever-existing, ever-conscious, ever-new bliss).

It is impossible to know and realize our true nature, the Self (the inner knower, which is self-existent) with our limited senses and intellect. The human mind, which is formed by thoughts, ideas, desires, memories and imagination is finite and cannot possibly fathom the infinite reality. The mind, being a subtle force of matter, creates its own world of experiences and relationships to objects according to its desire. Through desire, attachment, a sense of ego, ignorance and misidentification with the mind, body and senses, we experience suffering, pain and unhappiness. Through misidentification and forgetfulness of our true nature as spiritual beings we lose awareness of the Self, the very source of inner happiness, inner peace and inner joy.

As spiritual beings made in the likeness and image of God we are endowed with an innate capacity to completely awaken to and realize the pure bliss-consciousness of the soul and our conscious relationship with the infinite. Meditation awakens us to know and realize our true spiritual nature here and now. Through meditation we re-establish our true spiritual identity and remember our eternal loving relationship with God.

We realize through meditation that we are not the physical form, mind, intellect, ego or senses. We realize that heaven is within, that it is not a place that we go to after death, but a consciousness of God, that can be realized and experienced here and now in this moment. Meditation brings us to the realization that God is above and beyond the conception of the finite mind, that nothing exists outside Him, that in Him we live, move and have our being, and that nothing in this finite world can give us the inner security, inner strength, inner peace, inner joy, love, happiness, freedom, complete satisfaction and lasting fulfilment that is in Him. Meditation is the direct way to knowing and realizing that we are one with the Infinite.

THE MASTERS ON MEDITATION

The Kingdom of God is within you.
Jesus Christ, in Luke 17:21

The soul loves to meditate, for in contact with the spirit lies its greater joy. Remember this when you experience mental resistance during meditation. Reluctance to meditate comes from the ego. It doesn't belong to the soul.
Paramhansa Yogananda, from The Essence of Self-Realization by Sri Kriyananda

Self-realization is the aim of life. The means to it are living an ethical life and ceaseless meditation.
Swami Sivananda of Rishikesh

The greatest help to spiritual life is meditation. In meditation we divest ourselves of all material conditions and feel our divine nature. We do not depend upon any external help in meditation.
Swami Vivekanada, Teachings of Swami Vivekananda

We meditate not to attain God, but to perceive that God who is already attained.
Swami Muktananda

Meditate on Him alone, on Him, the Fountain of Goodness. Pray to Him; depend on Him. Try to give more time to japa and meditation. Surrender your mind at His feet.
Sri Anandamayi Ma

> *Real meditation is getting absorbed in God as the only thought, the only goal. God only, only God. Think God, breathe God, love God, live God.*
>
> Sathya Sai Baba, *Conversations*

THE PRACTICE OF MEDITATION

Where to Meditate

For your daily sitting meditation, it is important to choose a place which you will use regularly, and only for meditation. This will help to create a meditative vibration and a spiritual atmosphere in the place where you will sit.

The meditation place should be kept simple, clean and sacred. If possible, have a separate room and use it only for meditation. The other alternative is to either screen off a small section of a room or find a suitable corner or place in a room where you can sit regularly for meditation without being disturbed.

Wherever you decide to sit for your meditation make sure that it feels comfortable. It should be free from clutter, distractions, noise, pollution and other people. The temperature should be balanced so that you do not become drowsy with the heat or shivering with the cold. Try to have some fresh air circulating in the room by opening a window. This will help to keep you awake and alert during meditation.

Meditation Shrine

In your meditation area you may like to set up a small shrine or altar (an outer symbol of God-communion) on which you can place a picture or pictures of your spiritual Master, guru, Christ, Krishna, or saints that spiritually inspire you.

On the altar you can also place some fresh flowers in a vase of water, light a candle and burn either incense or pure essential oils. The flowers are an offering of your love and devotion to God and the gurus. The candlelight and incense or pure essential oils create a good ambience for meditation. The following pure essential oils are particularly good for meditation: sandalwood, frankincense, rose, rosewood, benzoin, cedarwood, myrrh and juniper.

Essential oils are flammable, so do not put them on or near a naked flame. The way to use them is to vaporize them. To do this you will need an aromatherapy burner or vaporizer. Float up to five drops of pure essential oils on water at the top of the bowl and light a small (night light) candle underneath to heat the water. As the oil evaporates it releases its aroma into the air, purifying the atmosphere and the mind. Some essential oils help to create a feeling of love, harmony and relaxation, while others spiritually uplift the consciousness and help to calm the conscious mind, inducing a mood that leads to meditation.

When you set up your altar and sit in front of it to meditate, have it positioned so that you face north or east. This is because the polarity of the magnetic fields of the Earth subtly influence us. Facing north or east will create a positive effect, while facing south will create a negative effect on the mind.

When to Meditate

It is important to establish a regular, fixed time for meditation, so that your mind and body become accustomed to it. Once you have established a time and place, be consistent.

The best times to meditate are at 6.00 am (sunrise), 12.00 noon, 6.00 pm (sunset) and 12.00 midnight. It is at these times that the gravitational pull of the sun works in harmony with the natural polarity of the body. If you cannot meditate at all these times then do so at sunrise and just before retiring to sleep at night.

In India, the yogis say that the most auspicious and peaceful time to meditate in the morning is between the early hours of 4.00 am and 6.00 am. This auspicious time is called *brahmamuhurta*. At this time there is the quality of peacefulness and goodness (*sattva*) predominant in the mind of the meditator and in the atmosphere. It is a time when most worldly people are asleep, so there are no distractions. There is a stillness in the atmosphere at this time that makes it particularly favourable for meditation. It is also at this time and at dusk that the energy in the *sushumna nadi* flows readily. You will know when the *sushumna nadi* is flowing, because the breath will be flowing equally through both nostrils.

If your aspiration for God and truth is sincere, then you will discipline yourself to meet your appointment with God in daily meditation at the same time every day. Remember God first; everything else can wait. When God comes first in your life, then it is easy to adjust your outer life to make time to meditate.

Length of Meditation

If you have not sat for meditation before, then sit for only five to ten minutes in the beginning. It is more important to develop the habit of meditating regularly than to sit for half an hour feeling bored and restless, or to sit for half an hour one day and then not meditate at all the next.

Be consistent and regular in your practice. Start with five- to ten-minute periods until you have strongly developed the habit of meditation, then gradually lengthen the periods to 15 minutes. If you can do this without creating any mental tension and can remain soulfully centred in a calm meditative state, then increase the length of your meditation to 20 minutes.

Sit for meditation twice daily, for 20 minutes. As you progress, gradually increase the length of each period. At weekends when you have more time, increase it to two or three times as long as your daily meditations. A 20-minute meditation can be increased to one hour. As you progress, you will experience that the more you meditate, the more you will want to meditate. Rapid progress and success in meditation depends on consistent, regular practice and your faith, sincerity, patience, perseverance, relaxed effort and interest.

Depth of Meditation

Both the Masters of yoga, Paramhansa Yogananda and Swami Sivananda of Rishikesh, instructed their disciples to increase their period of meditation gradually to three hours. This is what we should aim for if we want to attain the superconscious state of *samadhi*.

But more important than the length of time is the depth of meditation. Our meditation is wasted if we sit for three hours daydreaming or slip into a drowsy subconscious state. If this happens, then it is better to meditate for only 20 or 30 minutes with attentive concentration and alertness.

Achieving Deep Meditation

1 The body needs to be completely relaxed and remain motionless.
2 Stop stimulation from outside by internalizing the five senses.
3 The mind needs to be completely alert, attentively aware and internally focused.
4 All the scattered forces of the mind must be focused on a single point of concentration at the spiritual eye (the centre of will, intuition and superconsciousness). You need to lift your awareness into superconsciousness.
5 When the attention of the mind has been freed from all restlessness and is focused on God in a state of deep calmness, expansion of consciousness can be experienced through both devotion and inner communion. God can manifest Himself in eight primary ways: light, sound, power, wisdom, calmness, peace, love and joy. When you experience deep meditation and become absorbed in any of these qualities, then your consciousness becomes expanded and attuned to God.
6 Stick to one meditation method, or to those taught by your guru. Be patient, do not be a collector of different techniques and gurus. Stay with one meditation method and master it completely. Persevere, be regular and consistent for a long period of time.
7 Surrender your body, senses and mind-ego to God, for it is only by surrendering ourselves to God that we can realize Him. The moment we forget God, the ego reappears, so self-surrender is the result of a constant stream of God-remembrance. When the ego is conquered by self-surrender, the mind becomes still, and in the calm, still mind God reveals Himself.
8 Meditation on its own is not enough to please God. More than anything else He wants our undivided, loving attention. God will lovingly respond to us when we make an effort towards Him, by thinking of Him during our activities throughout the day, as well as in meditation.

When we can balance our outer activities in life with meditation, by right activity and remaining in the awareness of God's presence attained in meditation, then we will have deeper meditations.

Postures

The traditional yogic *asanas* (postures) for sitting meditation are the lotus pose (*padmasana*), the accomplished pose (*siddhasana*), the auspicious pose (*swastikasana*) and the easy pose (*sukhasana*). Buddhists and Zen meditators tend to sit in the thunderbolt pose (*vajrasana*). You can also sit in an upright chair for meditation, if for some reason you are unable to sit in a crossed-leg posture. A steady correct posture is essential for meditation, especially when it becomes deeper and longer. The chosen posture should allow you to sit steadily and comfortably, so that you can remain with the body still and relaxed for the duration of your meditation.

The spine, neck and head must remain straight but relaxed throughout the meditation. In this way the energies of the physical body are transmuted and the life-force (*prana*) is quickened and intensified as

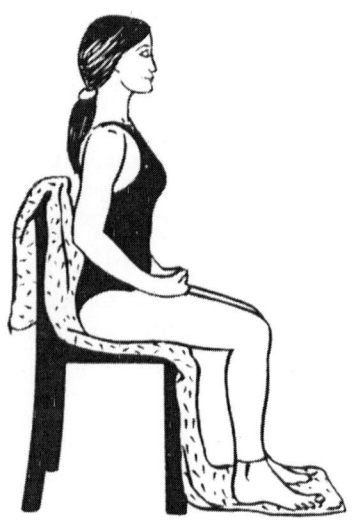

Figure 20 *Position for meditation seated on a chair*

energies are allowed to flow freely through the physical and subtle nerve systems. If you slump forward, with your spine bent, then you short-circuit the life-energies of your body.

1. The chair should be upright and armless, and should be covered by a woollen blanket. Allow enough blanket to flow onto the floor, so that you can insulate your feet and body against the earth's subtle magnetic currents, which tend to pull the mind towards material thoughts.
2. Sit upright, with your back away from the back of the chair. Keep your spine, head and neck in a straight line, but relaxed. Relax your hands and place them, palms upwards, at the junction of the thighs and abdomen to help keep the spine erect and the chest open. Your feet should be flat on the floor about hip-width apart.
3. If the seat of the chair is too hard, then sit on a folded blanket or cushion to make it more comfortable.

Sukhasana: The Easy Pose

This is a very basic and simple crossed-leg pose, good for beginners.

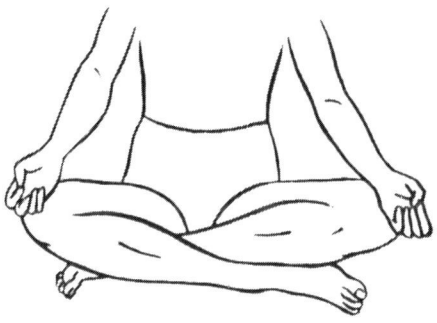

Figure 21 *Sukhasana*

1. Sit by folding your right foot under your left thigh and your left foot under your right thigh.
2. Place your hands, palms upwards, on the knees.
3. It is a good idea to sit on a folded blanket or cushion to take the strain out of your knees and lower back.

Swastikasana: The Auspicious Pose

If you find *padmasana* and *siddhasana* difficult you can practise *swastikasana*, especially if you are going to sit for a long meditation. But do *not* practise it if you are suffering from sciatica or sacral infections, or if you have torn or injured cartilages in the knees.

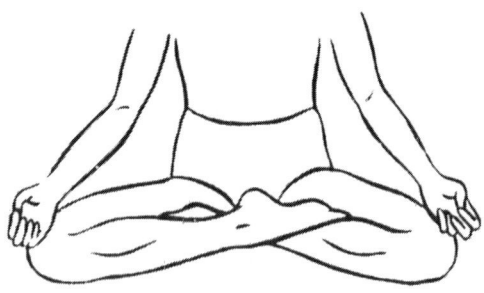

Figure 22 *Swastikasana*

1 Sit with your legs outstretched. Then bend your left leg and place the heel of your left foot against your right groin, with the sole of the foot touching the right thigh muscles.
2 Bend your right leg so that it crosses over the left and gently insert the toes of your right foot between your left thigh and calf muscles.
3 The toes of both feet should lie between the thighs and calves of the legs.
4 Keep your trunk, neck and head in a straight line.
5 Your hands can rest on the knees in *gyana* or *chin mudra* (see chapter 4), or they can rest one on top of the other, palms up in the lap.

Siddhasana: The Accomplished Pose

If you find *padmasana* difficult, practice *siddhasana*. This is a good posture for long, deep meditations. It is also good for control over the sexual function, which the yogi or meditator can either use to maintain celibacy by rechannelling the sexual energy upwards to the brain for spiritual purposes, or to gain greater control over the sensory sexual function.

Siddhasana tones the sexual glands and has a calming effect on the mind and the nervous system. It also directs *prana* into the *sushumna*.

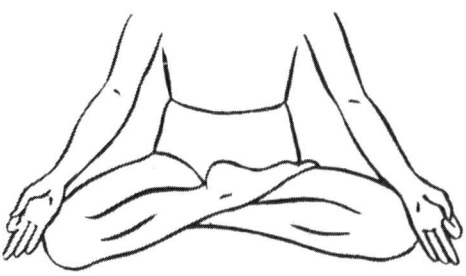

Figure 23 *Siddhasana*

1 Sit with your legs stretched forward.
2 Bend your left leg and place the heel of your left foot against the perineum (the area between the genitals and the anus).
3 Bend your right leg over the left and place your right foot on the left thigh with the right heel resting on the genitals, directly over the left heel. The legs should now be locked, with the knees on the ground.
4 Keep your trunk, neck and head in a straight line.
5 Place your hands on the knees in *gyana* or *chin mudra*.

This pose can be practised in combination with the three *bandhas* (see chapter 4). But do *not* practise it if you suffering from sciatica, sacral infections or torn or injured knee cartilages.

Siddha Yoni Asana: The Female Accomplished Pose

This pose was devised for women by Swami Satyananda Saraswati. It has a direct effect on the nerve plexuses which control the female reproductive system and gives control over the neuro-psychic impulses which are used by the yogi for spiritual purposes.

It is basically the same as *siddhasana* but it differs in so much as the heel of the lower foot is pressed inside the labia majora of the vagina. It is best done without underwear on.

Padmasana: The Lotus Pose

The lotus is a beautiful flower that symbolizes beauty, peace and purity.

Padmasana is the most advanced of the sitting postures. If you look at pictures of great yogis and Masters, such as Mahavatar Babaji, Lahiri Mahasaya, Swami Sri Yukteswar and Paramhansa Yogananda, you will see that they are all sitting in *padmasana*. For most Westerners it is a difficult posture to get into, particularly for those adults whose legs are stiff from years of sedentary living.

Before attempting this posture it is advisable to practise leg warm-up exercises, particularly for the knee joints. From my own experience in damaging a knee cartilage by practising the lotus pose, I advise you to be extremely careful when practising this pose.

Here are some guidelines:

- Make sure your legs, knees and ankle joints are warm. If they are cold and stiff, then you will need to do some warming-up exercises.
- Never force the knees into the lotus position, as you may tear the knee ligaments, which can be very painful! Practise slowly, gradually and very carefully.
- Take time to warm up and relax your legs and knees. You can relax the knees by rubbing the sides vigorously with your palms. By doing this the bursae lubricate and protect the knees from forcible flexion.
- Loosen up the hips, knees and pelvic girdle with warm-up stretches.

The technique is as follows:
1. Sit with your legs extended forward and align your whole body.
2. Bend your right leg slowly and carefully over the left (keeping the muscles of the leg relaxed), bringing the thigh in and taking the right foot into the groin. Keep your left leg well extended, especially in the knee joint.
3. Now bring your right knee closer to your left groin.
4. Bend your left leg and place the foot in front of your right shin (as you do this hold your left heel with your right hand and your left ankle with your left hand).
5. Raise your left foot by the ankle and place it into the right groin, so that the legs are now crossed. You can bring the knees closer together.

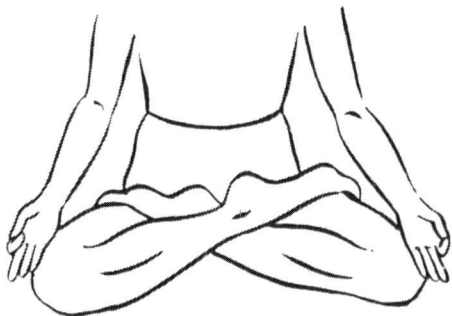

Figure 24 Padmasana (lotus pose)

6 Keep your trunk, neck and head straight but relaxed.
7 Place your hands on your knees in *gyana* or *chin mudra*, or with the relaxed palms facing upwards, one on top of the other, in your lap.

Padmasana increases the blood supply to the visceral organs, tones the coccygeal and sacral nerves, and stimulates the digestive system. It directs the flow of *prana* from the *muladhara chakra* to the *sahasrara chakra*. It calms the mind and gives a perfect sense of psychosomatic equilibrium. It also gives flexibility to the hips, knees and ankles.

It should *not* be practised by people with sciatica, sacral infections or torn or injured cartilages.

Ardha Padmasana: Half-lotus Pose

This posture is a good preparation for the full lotus.

1 Sit with your legs outstretched in front of you.
2 Bend your left leg and place the left foot beside the right thigh.
3 Bend your right leg and place the right foot on top of the left thigh.
4 Keep your trunk, neck and head in a straight line.
5 Place the hands on the knees in *gyana mudra*.

Do *not* practise this if you are suffering from sciatica, sacral infections or torn or injured cartilages.

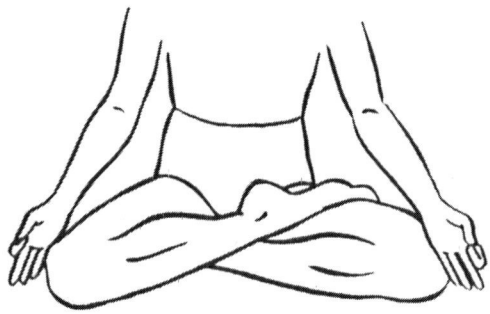

Figure 25 *Ardha padmasana*

When you have mastery in *asana* and you are able to sit steady in your posture, then you will not be distracted by the body or even feel the body when you sit for meditátion.

To make your *asana* more comfortable, place one or two cushions or folded blankets beneath your buttocks. This raises the buttocks and lowers the knees towards the floor, easing any tension there might be in the knees and lower back.

WAKING EARLY FOR MORNING MEDITATION

For many beginners, meditation can be a struggle, and there can be many obstacles to overcome before the regular and consistent practice of meditation is successfully established in one's life.

One of the main reasons for not rising early and enthusiastically in the morning to meditate is that sincere interest may be lacking. The mind-ego does not want to meditate, it does not want to be disciplined and so it always makes excuses to avoid it. The ego is cunning. When you are awoken by the alarm clock, you open your eyes and the mind says 'Oh my God, it's six o'clock, I should be meditating; I'm so tired, I'll just have another five minutes' sleep, then get up.' But before you know it, you have slept not five minutes, but an hour. It is now 7.00 am and you have missed your appointment with God!

The following guidelines will help you rise early for meditation.

- **Develop a sincere, conscious interest and aspiration to want to know and realize God**. What is needed is enthusiasm, persistent effort and urgency. Very few people have this urgency. It is something that cannot be learned from somebody, or taught, it must develop from within oneself.
- **Practise self-inquiry and contemplate the importance of meditation**. Ask yourself: 'How can I know and realize God?' 'What is life? What is death? What happens to us after death?' 'What is God?' 'What is "I"?' 'What is the nature of the mind?' 'What is bliss?' 'How can the restless, rebellious mind be made calm and serene?' 'What is the aim of yoga and meditation?' 'What do the great gurus and Masters say about meditation?'
- **Make an appointment with God**. In our hearts we know that God takes first place within our lives, because without God life is meaningless and there is always that feeling that something is missing from our lives. God, who is love, is seated within our hearts, but most of us have forgotten Him and as a result feel an emptiness within. To experience God's love, joy, peace and wisdom, and realize His presence within us we need to remember Him – keep Him foremost in our thoughts – and surrender the ego. The first thought that arises every morning is the 'I' thought (the observer, the knower, the doer). This thought then connects itself to and assumes ownership of the other thoughts that stream forth from the mind. The first 'I' thought, simultaneously as it arises, casts behind itself a shadow of ignorance.

  Replace your first thoughts of the morning ('I don't want to meditate', 'I'm tired', 'I would rather sleep than meditate', etc) with 'God first'! Affirm positively:

  > I attune my thoughts and activities to God's unfailing presence and power. God's Will is my will. I will meditate and let God work in and through my mind and heart so that I can express divine qualities. I begin my day in communication with God: through meditation I bring an attitude of harmony to all that I do today. Centred in God, my thoughts and activities are God directed.

- **Eliminate toxins and stimulants and eat lightly at night**. Eating heavy, hard-to-digest, stimulating foods at night keeps the heart and lungs hard at work digesting food. To sleep properly one must be able to withdraw the energy from the muscles, organs and conscious mind. Eat lightly in the evenings and try not to eat any later than 6.00 pm. Choose vegetarian foods that help your mind maintain its tranquillity, alertness and clarity. The body will then retain its vitality and the mind will be clear and elevated for the evening meditation and afterwards sleep.

Avoid stimulating and spicy foods at night (garlic, onions, spices, sugar, salt). Eliminate all stimulating beverages. The caffeine in coffee and the bromine in tea have an adverse effect on the nervous system. Caffeine is particularly stimulating to the adrenal glands, and interferes with the quality of your sleep. Alcohol artificially relaxes, but when the effects wear off, the body is left feeling heavy and the mind is usually dulled and depressed. Other drinks to avoid, especially at night, are colas, cocoa and chocolate.

- **Avoid stimulating activities at night.** As we approach evening meditation time and afterwards sleep, we need to prepare by relaxing the muscles and organs of the body. We need to calm the mind and nervous system. For the mind to be serene we should avoid reading the newspapers and watching television, as any stimulating or disturbing news or programmes may disturb or agitate the mind, making it tense or restless. Be selective in what you watch, hear and read, if you want to keep a serene mind, have a quality sleep and rise early for meditation. Avoid arguments, heated debates and excessive talking. Keep silence late at night.
- **Relax the mind and body.** Practise a few yoga postures slowly with awareness and alternate nostril breathing. Then practise complete relaxation with awareness as you lie in *shavasana* (as in the practice of *yoga nidra* – see chapter 7). You will then feel relaxed and refreshed to sit and meditate. Afterwards when you retire to bed, you will have a quality sleep.

    The yoga postures eliminate stress and tension from the muscles by gently squeezing and stretching them. They also harmonize the subtle energy currents in the body, allowing you to relax completely.
- **Affirm that you will wake early.** The subconscious mind is receptive to suggestions and affirmations just before falling asleep. So with conscious conviction and deep concentration on the spiritual eye, repeat the following affirmation, first aloud, then whisper it,

then repeat it mentally with feeling, lifting the consciousness aspiringly toward superconsciousness.

As I rest and sleep, I am renewed with new energy and vitality, I will awake early at six o'clock, positive, energetic and enthusiastic for meditation.

You can then end your affirmation by offering it up to God in loving prayer:

Divine Mother, awaken me early for meditation. Awaken my love for Thee and help me to think of Thee first.

The best time for morning meditation is between the hours of 4.00 am and 6.00 am, *brahmamuhurta* (the hour of God). To meditate at this time you will need to go to bed by 9.00 or 10.00 the night before. You will probably need at least six hours' sleep. As you progress and deepen your meditation, and as you meditate regularly, you will be able to reduce the number of hours you sleep. Paramhansa Yogananda would only sleep for two or three hours, as do other very advanced yogis and gurus.

There are many people who are sleeping their lives away. Those who are living a healthy life, practising yoga, *pranayama* and meditation should not be sleeping more than six hours. Time and energy is wasted in sleeping 7–12 hours. For a yogi, much of this time is better utilized in meditation. Also, it is not how many hours you have slept that is important, but how restful your sleep is. A yogi who knows the art of sleeping and *yoga nidra* can actually decide by will when he returns to normal consciousness and aspiration. The nights are used by advanced yogis to continue their *sadhana* (spiritual practice).

As an exercise in waking at will, you can train the subconscious mind to wake you at fixed intervals throughout the night. Allow three hours for the first interval. Just before falling asleep consciously affirm as you look into the spiritual eye, that you *will* wake at 2.00 am, returning to your normal consciousness and aspiration for God. In this exercise do not use an alarm. Then consciously affirm and will yourself to wake at the next interval, which could be at 3.00 am. Then return to sleep consciously relaxing the mind and body, knowing that God, who is love, is seated within your heart. Surrender yourself to this love within you.

Thoughts Arising in Meditation

Without deep concentration of mind you cannot meditate. A mind that is restless with wandering thoughts will divert your attention away from the object of meditation. Meditation is an uninterrupted, unceasing flow of attentive awareness and concentration on God. It is like the smooth, unbroken continuity of oil being poured into one spot.

The mind in meditation can be compared to a glass of muddy water. If the water is agitated, it will become very cloudy with particles of dirt. If we want it to look more transparent and clear, then we must leave it undisturbed, so that the particles of dirt sink back to the bottom of the glass, allowing the water to become clear.

The mind can also be compared to the ocean, with the rising thoughts and emotions like waves on the ocean. In its natural state the ocean is calm. It is only when some turbulence is caused by a storm, the wind or strong undercurrents that waves arise. When the storm subsides, the waves merge back into the calm ocean.

So when countless thought waves and emotions arise in the mind during meditation, do not invite them in, pursue them, or identify with them. Make no effort to fight or control them. Allow the thoughts to arise and settle back into the mind from where they came. As each thought arises be aware of it, then effortlessly let it return to the mind, without any involvement in it.

Thought is the nature of mind. To transcend thought and quieten the mind, what is required is an understanding independent of thought, a direct awareness of the movements of the mind.

It is necessary to recognize the distraction of thoughts without being absorbed in them. The pure consciousness, which is your true Self, is not the transitory thoughts of which it is aware, but the silent witness behind all thoughts.

When a thought arises in your mind, ask to whom the thought has arisen. Whose thought is it? Where does it arise from? Then ask, 'Who am I?'

If the body and mind are not properly prepared for meditation, then there will be many distractions, both physical and mental. To prepare for meditation, the body must be comfortable, relaxed and still, otherwise the mind will become restless. We can prepare the body through the practice of Hatha Yoga, by loosening up the spine, hips, knees and ankle joints. Yoga postures, and in particular, *pranayama* (see chapter 5), will greatly aid in relaxing and calming the mind. Once the mind is freed from mental tensions, worries and anxieties, we then withdraw its attention and the senses from the objects of sense by closing out the outward causes of distraction and internalizing the life-force. When the mind is disconnected from the senses, abstraction of the senses (*pratyahara*) follows automatically. Dispassion and renunciation are very helpful in the practice of *pratyahara*. One who can discipline the mind and senses perfectly attains inner strength, strong will, perfect concentration and peace of mind.

The mind is then given an object to concentrate on (mantra, chakra, inner light, inner sound, breath), so that it can be absorbed with that one object to the exclusion of everything else. When the mind is quiet and still, the conscious awareness of the truth of our being is revealed.

THE *BHAGAVAD GITA*'S INSTRUCTION ON MEDITATION

In the *Bhagavad Gita*, Lord Krishna gives spiritual instructions on the practice of meditation:

> *Free from ever-expecting desires and attachments, with the body and mind controlled, the yogi should seek to know the inner Self through meditation, in solitude.*
>
> *Having found a clean place that is neither too high nor too low, and having placed a firm seat first with kusha grass, then a deerskin, followed by a cloth, sit firmly on this seat. Then with the mind and senses under control, concentrate with one-pointed attention on the subject of meditation to purify the heart.*
>
> *Holding the trunk, head and neck straight and steady, remaining still and freeing the eyes from distraction, concentrate the gaze at the point between the eyebrows.*
>
> *Established in the calmness of the Self, undisturbed by fears, firmly resolved in brahmacharya, with the mind controlled and absorbed in Me, the yogi should sit in meditation with Me as the ultimate goal.*
>
> *The yogis who ceaselessly practise control of the body, mind and senses attain the eternal peace of My being, consisting of supreme bliss, which has its foundation in Me.*
>
> Bhagavad Gita 6: 10–15

The Basic Procedure and Technique for Meditation

1 **Clean the body.** Take a warm shower followed by a quick cold shower to clean and enliven the body. Cleanliness of the body and the place where you sit for meditation is important for the purification of the consciousness.
2 **Energize and relax the body.** Awaken the body and brain cells by recharging them with energy. In meditation it is particularly important to increase the flow of pranic energy to the spine, so that it can be raised to the higher brain centres. By withdrawing the life-force from the senses and centring it in the spine, then directing it upward through the spine to the brain and the spiritual eye the consciousness can merge in the infinite consciousness.

    Paramhansa Yogananda taught his disciples a systematic method called the 'energization exercises'. They were developed to increase the flow of life-force to every part of the body at will, to energize, heal and strengthen it. I practise these energization exercises myself as a devotee of Yogananda and have experienced the benefit of this direct energy flowing into my body. They definitely recharge the body with energy when practised with an attitude of willingness, and with an inner awareness.

    Those yoga students who feel drawn to the path of Kriya Yoga and would like to learn the energization exercises, should write to the Ananda Church of Self-realization, whose address is given at the end of the book.

    You can also energize the body by practising a few *asanas* before meditation. As you perform them with awareness, concentrate on the flow of energy in the spine. There are certain postures, such as *maha mudra* (see chapter 4), *bhujangasana* (see below), *viparita karani mudra* (see chapter 4) and *dhanurasana* (see below) that help in increasing the flow of energy in the spine. The yoga postures also help to release stress and relax the body in preparation for meditation.
3 **Sit with a correct posture.** With the body and mind relaxed, sit upright with your head, neck and spine in a straight line. Your body should be comfortable and relaxed. Be aware of your natural breath and the flow of energy in the spine.
4 **Quieten the mind.** If your mind is constantly restless, like a monkey jumping from tree to tree, you will find it very difficult to

Bhujangasana (cobra pose)

Method:
1. Lie face down on the floor, arms by your sides, forehead resting on the floor, and your feet about 30 cms (1 ft) apart.
2. Bend your elbows and place your hands under your shoulders.
3. Inhale, and slowly raise your head and neck first, followed by your chest. Drop and relax your shoulders as you come up. Look straight ahead.
4. Slowly, rise up into the full cobra pose, by extending your arms and arching your spine and neck backwards. Keep your feet, legs and hips on the floor. Raise your sternum and top ribs and pull your shoulders back and down, away from your ears.
   Hold the position for 10–20 seconds, breathing evenly. Advanced students can increase the period up to one minute.
5. To come out of the pose, exhale and gradually lower your body to the floor by first lowering your abdomen, then your chest, neck and head. Relax. Repeat the practice up to five times.

Caution: Do not practise if you have:
- peptic ulcer
- hernia

Benefits:
- It gives flexibility to the spine, expands the chest and ribcage.
- It is good for asthma and respiratory problems.
- It stimulates and massages the nerves and muscles of the spine.
- It tones the ovaries and uterus in women.
- It is beneficial for the liver and kidneys.

Dhanurasana (the bow)

Method:
1. Lie down on the front of your body, with your forehead resting on the floor.

2 Bend your knees and grasp your ankles with your hands. Allow your knees to be slightly apart.
3 Inhale and raise your head, chest and thighs off the ground as high as possible; so that your body is resting on the abdomen.
4 Hold your breath for three deep breaths while holding the pose.
5 Exhale as you lower your body down and relax.
6 Repeat twice more. Try 'rocking' backwards and forwards in the final pose to massage the abdomen.

Benefits:
This is an excellent *asana* to massage and invigorate all the internal organs.
Tones up the abdominal muscles.
Regulates the pancreas, liver and spleen.
Gives flexibility to the spine.
Good for people who have diabetes.

Caution: This posture should not be practised by pregnant women.

make progress in your meditation. It is important to make the mind calm and quiet; if you can do this even for ten minutes you will make some progress. In meditation the mind is silent but is also consciously aware.

The practice of *pranayama* will help to quieten the mind. When the breath is restless, the mind also becomes unsteady, but when the breath is steady or still, so is the activity of the mind.

Practise nine rounds of *loma pranayama* (see chapter 5). This is a three-part equal-breath ratio, breathing through the nostrils. Inhale for six, retain for six, exhale for six (6: 6: 6). You can also practise *nadi shuddhi* (alternate nostril breathing – see chapter 5). This *pranayama* will help your meditation by soothing the nervous system and balancing the flow of breath in each nostril. When the flow is equal, *prana* begins to flow in the central main *nadi* (*sushumna*).

5 **Chant and pray.** Before you begin your meditation, chant the mantra *om* three times and offer prayers of devotion and love to God and the saints or gurus who inspire you. Pray for their grace, for

attunement, for the awareness of the presence of God, that you will be guided into deep meditation and inner communion with God. In prayer we seek to draw closer to God, to attract His grace. Pray in the language of your heart and open to the awareness of God's presence.

Your prayer can be followed by devotional chanting or singing to awaken your love and devotion for God. When we sing and chant the Names of God with sincerity and devotion from the heart, it creates energy, love and joy within us. With this devotional aspiration the energy is awakened in the spine; the mind becomes quiet and love and devotion well up in our hearts.

Begin your chanting aloud to awaken the energy within, then chant softly, becoming more inward by chanting in a whisper, then mentally with the aspiration of heart and soul.

6 **Concentrate.** Continue sitting upright and relaxed with your eyes closed. Remain still and concentrate your relaxed attention on the point between the eyebrows. Let go of all thoughts. Be totally centred in the present moment, here and now.

Keep your awareness on the natural breath as you continue to look into the spiritual eye. If your mind wanders, gently bring it back to the practice of watching the breath with awareness. Interiorize your mind by deepening your concentration until you become completely absorbed.

7 **Practise the *hong sau* technique.** This technique is described in chapter 7.

8 **Meditate – enter the secret door to infinity.** Continue the *hong sau* breath until the mind is calmly interiorized in deep concentration. Then go beyond the awareness of all techniques into the surrendered, receptive state of 'being'. Remain in the silent, deep, calm peace of the soul for as long as possible.

With your mind and heart surrendered in God, dissolve the boundaries of ego-consciousness (your sense of individuality and separateness) like a bubble dissolving in the cosmic sea. Feel and experience yourself as pure consciousness without name and form. Become one with the object of your meditation.

Deepen your awareness of God's presence within you by listening to the divine inner sounds (such as *om*), by gazing inwardly through the spiritual eye into the light, by experiencing inner joy, inner peace and divine love.

In this state of deep inner calm and silence, know that God is omnipresent and within you. Let that feeling of devotion and aspiration pour love into your mind, your heart and your whole being, until every cell in your body is vibrating with love and joy.

9 **Conclude your meditation.** Finish your meditation with a prayer for inner guidance in your life, for those who are close to you, and for world peace. Feel your mind and body to be purified, energized and in harmony with life and the universe.

10 **Remain centred after meditation.** Remain calmly centred within as you go about your regular everyday activities with willingness and purpose, knowing that you are in the presence of God and that your life is being guided inwardly by the divine intelligence.

AFFIRMATION

Every day, I set aside time to commune with God. As I enter into the meditative silence, I release all thoughts, problems, worries and anxieties. I rest within, in the peace of God.

Meditation restores order, balance and harmony to my life. In the stillness of my meditation I listen intuitively to the still inner voice of wisdom. I receive guidance and divine inspiration. All doubts and challenges are resolved. The seemingly impossible becomes possible. Through meditation my energy is renewed and my outlook is positive, energetic and enthusiastic.

KRIYA YOGA: AN ADVANCED SPIRITUAL ACCELERATOR

The ancient and advanced techniques of Kriya Yoga meditation were first revealed to the great Master, Lahiri Mahasaya by his great Master, Mahavatar Babaji in 1861. Before 1861, this sacred science was inaccessible to the world. Lahiri Mahasaya had obtained permission from Babaji to impart it to all sincerely seeking souls.

Kriya Yoga was passed down to a disciplic succession of great

Masters (who were all avatars) in the following order: Mahavatar Babaji, Lahiri Mahasaya, Swami Sri Yukteswar. Paramhansa Yogananda was the last Master in this particular line of gurus, who left his body in *mahasamadhi* (departure from the physical body in superconscious communion with God) in 1952.

Lahiri Mahasaya (1828–95) initiated some 5,000 disciples into Kriya in India. Swami Sri Yukteswar (1855–1936, initiated by his guru Lahiri Mahasaya in 1883) and Paramhansa Yogananda (1893–1952) also initiated thousands of devotees into the sacred meditation.

Lahiri Mahasaya and Sri Yukteswar had their own lineage of realized disciples, who were permitted to initiate others into the holy science of Kriya.

Paramhansa Yogananda was the only Kriya Master who set up a formal Kriya Yoga organization, called the Self-Realization Fellowship.

In 1920 the great Babaji instructed Yogananda to spread the message of Kriya Yoga to the West.

Kriya Yoga, the scientific technique of God-realization, will ultimately spread in all lands and aid in harmonizing the nations through man's personal, transcendental perception of the Infinite Father.

Paramhansa Yogananda, *Autobiography of a Yogi*

Deeply touched by these words Yogananda left his beloved guru's ashram and India in 1920 to begin his spiritual mission of teaching Kriya Yoga in the West. Part of his mission was also to demonstrate the underlying unity between the teachings of India, as expressed in the *Bhagavad Gita*, and the original teachings of Christ as given in the Bible. Yogananda showed that all religions, whatever their outward forms, are rooted in the same essential truth.

WHAT IS KRIYA YOGA?

The Kriya Yoga which I am giving to the world through you in this 19th century [Babaji told Lahiri Mahasaya] is a revival of the same science which Krishna gave, millenniums ago, to Arjuna, and which was later known to Patanjali and to Christ, St John, St Paul and other disciples.

Mahavatar Babaji, from *Autobiography of a Yogi* by **Paramhansa Yogananda**

> *Meditate unceasingly, that you may quickly behold yourself as the infinite essence, free from every form of misery. Cease being a prisoner of the body; using the secret key of Kriya, learn to escape into spirit.*
>
> Lahiri Mahasaya, ibid

> *Kriya Yoga is an instrument through which human evolution can be quickened.*
>
> Swami Sri Yukteswar, ibid

> *Kriya, controlling the mind directly through the life-force, is the easiest, most effective, and most scientific avenue of approach to the infinite.*
>
> Paramhansa Yogananda, ibid

The Sanskrit word *Kriya* means 'to do', 'action', and *yoga* means 'union'. Kriya Yoga therefore means a certain action or active process to achieve the science of uniting the soul with God.

Kriya Yoga is the essence of all yogas. It is an effective and direct approach to God-realization. Through the correct and regular practice of Kriya Yoga meditation, with love and devotion for God, the *kriyaban* or Kriya yogi in an expanded state of consciousness can have a direct experience of the omnipresent love and bliss of the Divine.

Kriya Yoga meditation awakens subtle currents of energy in the spine and higher brain centres. With the spine and brain magnetized with energy the Kriya yogi consciously directs the life-force upwards through the spine and brain to the spiritual eye, where the yogi meditates on the inner sound and inner light to expand his or her consciousness into cosmic consciousness.

> *The Kriya yogi mentally directs his life energy to revolve, upward and downward, around the six spinal centres (medullary, cervical, dorsal, lumbar, sacral and coccygeal plexuses) which correspond to the twelve astral signs of the zodiac, the symbolic cosmic man. One half-minute of revolution of energy around the sensitive spinal cord of man effects subtle progress in his evolution; that half-minute of kriya equals one year of natural spiritual unfoldment.*
>
> Paramhansa Yogananda, *Autobiography of a Yogi*

The Kriya Yoga meditation techniques are not given in this book, because it is the tradition of the Kriya Masters that these techniques will not be revealed to those who are curiosity seekers or 'just wanting to try them out'. The path of Kriya requires a long-term commitment.

Kriya carries with it the blessings of the great God-realized Masters who are gurus of this path – Jesus Christ, Babaji, Lahiri Mahasaya, Sri Yukteswar and Paramhansa Yogananda. Souls of this stature come only rarely into the world, and then as direct representatives of God sent to help uplift mankind. Through them and through the practice of Kriya Yoga will come into the world a great blessing or, as Yogananda called it, 'a new dispensation'.

REQUIREMENTS FOR KRIYA YOGA INITIATION

The path of Kriya Yoga includes the techniques of energization, *hong sau* and *aum*, which should be practised regularly every day for several months before initiation. On average, it takes about one year to prepare. The requirements for Kriya initiation at Ananda, whom I represent as the Ananda meditation group leader in London, are summarized below.

1 **Basic information.** If you have not already read Paramhansa Yogananda's *Autobiography of a Yogi* and Kriyananda's *The Path*, this will be your first step. After reading these books, you should re-read the chapter in each called 'Kriya Yoga'. These words of wisdom will continue to inspire you for as long as you practise Kriya.
2 **Discipleship.** You should feel an attitude of discipleship toward the line of Kriya Yoga Masters: Jesus Christ, Babaji-Krishna, Lahiri Mahasaya, Sri Yukteswar, and Paramhansa Yogananda. You should also particularly wish to receive Kriya Yoga initiation through Ananda. It is best to come to the Kriya initiation as a disciple of this path already. To this end Kriyananda has created a discipleship initiation ceremony which is given frequently at Ananda Village, Ananda World Brotherhood colonies, or wherever Ananda ministers are travelling. Discipleship initiation is a requirement for Kriya Yoga initiation.
3 **Meditation.** Because Kriya is a technique of meditation, by the time of your initiation you will need to have established a regular discipline of meditating already, usually for not less than one and a half hours daily. This is time of *silent meditation* and does not include

time spent in practices such as energization, yoga postures, or chanting, although all of these practices are certainly valuable in augmenting the quality of the time spent in silent, still meditation. This hour and a half can be divided into shorter periods, such as 30 or 45 minutes twice or thrice daily. Your *sadhana* (spiritual practices) should include daily practice of the major techniques of this path, given below.

- *Energization exercises.* You should have a thorough knowledge of how to do the exercises, as well as an understanding of the principles underlying them. Master tells us that these exercises are the 'cornerstone of this path'. They should be practised at least once, and preferably twice a day. (The energization technique is available through video and audio tapes, as well as a poster, but it is preferable to learn it in person from an Ananda minister.)
- *Hong sau technique.* This meditation technique of concentration, by which the mind is focused and brought into a state of peace should be practised daily. About six months after starting to practise this technique, one is eligible to receive discipleship initiation (see above) and the *aum* technique. (The *hong sau* technique is available in the correspondence course, *Lessons in Yoga: 14 Steps to Higher Awareness*, through a two-part video, *A Course in Meditation*, or directly from an Ananda minister.)
- *Aum technique.* This is a very high and sacred technique of meditation. The *aum* technique must be learned *in person* from an Ananda minister, usually at the same time you receive discipleship initiation. The *aum* technique should be added to your practice of energization and *hong sau* and all three techniques should be included as a regular part of your daily spiritual practices, for at least six months before you take the Kriya Yoga initiation.

4 **Study.** A study of Yogananda's and Kriyananda's teachings is very important. To take Kriya initiation through Ananda, it is required that you should have read Yogananda's *Autobiography of a Yogi.* You also need to have read Kriyananda's book, *The Path, A Spiritual Autobiography*, his booklet on discipleship, *A New Dispensation* and have studied his *Lessons in Yoga: 14 Steps to Higher Awareness.* We also highly recommend that you study other material about our path.

5 **The Ananda Church of God–realization.** Joining the Ananda Church of God–realization is a vehicle for your ongoing connection with Yogananda's ray of inspiration as it expresses itself through Kriyananda and the Ananda family. In addition to the Kriya ministry, the Church directs Ananda's worldwide work. You will receive continued support and inspiration through the Church newsletter, letters from Kriyananda and calls from Ananda ministers.
6 **Application.** After you have begun working towards fulfilling the above requirements, you may apply to the Kriya Ministry Office for initiation. Once you have filled out the application form, it is carefully reviewed and you are advised by letter, telephone or personal interview when you may take Kriya initiation, or what further steps are necessary to become eligible.
7 **Commitment.** You should realize that initiation into Kriya is only the first step in a lifelong commitment to this path. In order to continue to deepen your practice, you should have your Kriya practice checked at least twice a year by a qualified Kriya Yoga minister and attend retreats and group practice sessions for *kriyabans*.

A five-day Kriya preparation course is offered several times a year at Ananda's guest facility, The Expanding Light. Although it is not required, this course is highly recommended for all seeking Kriya initiation. We review the preliminary techniques (energization, *hong sau* and *aum*) as well as learning special Kriya preparation techniques. There is also time for personal retreat and silence. Kriya initiation is offered at the end of the course for those who have been approved by an Ananda Kriya minister.

Kriya Initiation at Ananda

Kriyananda, a direct disciple of Paramhansa Yogananda, was ordained by Yoganandaji in 1949 to conduct Kriya Yoga initiations, and he has continued to do so in the years since. In recent years, he has felt guided by Yogananda to designate Jyotish (John Novak) and Jaya (John Helin) to give the initiation as well. Kriya initiation is given by Ananda Kriya ministers at Ananda Village nearly every month and occasionally at other places such as Assisi in Italy, Seattle, Washington and Portland,

Oregon in the USA the American east coast and elsewhere. Information about specific times, dates and places is available on request.

Ongoing Support

A steady, dynamic practice of Kriya is helped by fellowship with other *kriyabans*, renewal of the Kriya vow, and regular reviews of your technique. As a part of our ministry services, we have a full-time Kriya minister to help you prepare for initiation and to support you in your continuing practice. In each of the Ananda World Brotherhood colonies (Sacramento, Palo Alto, Seattle, Portland, Austin and Assisi) there are ministers available to answer your questions and help you with your Kriya practice. Also, there are monthly guided *kriyaban* meditations at Ananda Village and the Ananda colonies.

Kriya lessons, tapes, a quarterly Kriyaban newsletter, and a Kriyaban library are available for all Ananda initiates through the Church office. Every June Kriyananda leads a special three-day *kriyaban* retreat. Several hundred initiates attend each year to receive inspiration, renew their Kriya vows, review their technique with specially trained ministers and meditate with other *kriyabans*.

For more information about Ananda and the addresses of the Ananda communities see Useful Addresses at the end of this book.

9

SAMADHI

Now we come to the attainment of the highest state of consciousness and true goal of life.

When the consciousness of the duality of subject and object disappears and only the true nature of the object contemplated remains, that is absorption (samadhi).

The Yoga Sutras of Patanjali 3:3

THE DIFFERENCE BETWEEN MEDITATION (DHYANA) AND SAMADHI

In meditation there is a *continuous* and *uninterrupted* flow of attention towards the object of meditation, whereas in *samadhi* there is a dissolution of the subjective/objective duality of consciousness of observer and observed. The mind is no longer conscious of itself as it merges with the object of meditation. Body consciousness also vanishes.

In meditation there is a succession of identical thought waves towards the object of meditation, but when meditation culminates in the enlightened state of *samadhi*, the meditator loses his or her individuality (ego-consciousness); expansion of consciousness and absorption begins. Beyond the mind, time and space, the individual consciousness of the meditator becomes totally absorbed and completely identified with the Absolute, the all-pervading, nameless, formless cosmic consciousness, in which all sense of duality completely disappears.

Here is a simplified example. When the attention is limited to a particular focal point, that is concentration (*dharana*); when it is continually flowing there, it is meditation (*dhyana*). For example, if I keep looking at you, it is concentration. When I am completely absorbed in looking at you, it is meditation. If I go deeper, these three (I–looking–you) become one, so that it is as though you alone are the reality and 'I' is non-existent; that is *samadhi*.

Since my whole consciousness is filled with this object to such an extent that I do not exist, that object alone exists fully and truly, I *know* that object intimately, immediately, in its complete essence. Remember the story of the boy who meditated on the buffalo. He lost his individuality and became one with the buffalo.

The Stages of *Samadhi*

Raja Yoga divides *samadhi* into two main categories:

- *samprajnata samadhi*, also known as *sa-bija samadhi* – 'with support' or 'with seed'
- *asamprajnata samadhi*, also known as *nir-bija samadhi* – 'without support' or 'seedless' – and *nirodha samadhi* – total control and final cessation of mental fluctuations (*vrittis*)

The difference between *samprajnata samadhi* and *asamprajnata samadhi* is that in *samprajnata* the mind needs an objective support (*alambana*) to meditate on whether gross (*vitarka*) or subtle (*vichara*), until the final state of *samprajnata (dharma–megha samadhi)* is attained. *Asamprajnata* has no objective support (*niralambana*).

> Samprajnata, *the* samadhi *of wisdom, occurs through the accompaniment of logical reasoning, contemplation, bliss, and the sense of pure being, 'I-am-ness'*
>
> *In* asamprajnata samadhi *there is a cessation of all mental activities, and the mind-stuff retains only unmanifested impressions.*
>
> The Yoga Sutras of Patanjali 1:17–18

> *One who is able to maintain a constant state of desirelessness, even towards the highest state of enlightenment, and maintains the highest discrimination and awareness attains* dharma-megha samadhi, *the cloud which showers the rain of divine virtue and heavenly grace.*
>
> *From that results freedom from afflictions (*kleshas*) (which cause pain and sorrow) and actions (*karmas*).*
>
> Ibid 4:29–30

The Lower Stages of *Samprajnata* (The *Samadhi* of Wisdom)

Patanjali describes the four types of *samprajnata samadhi* as '*vitarka–vicharanandasmita–rupanugamat–samprajnata*'.

Ibid 1:17

The names of these *samprajnata* are contained within the first two words of the sutra.

1 **Vitarka (savitarka and nirvitarka samadhi)**. *Savitarka samadhi* is the lowest *samadhi*, tainted by ignorance (*avidya*). The primary object of concentration is on the word-object-idea of gross physical forms (the five gross elements) and objects knowable through the senses.

 At the stage of *nirvitarka samadhi*, there is a transcendental direct perception of the object of concentration. There is no word-object-idea from the memory superimposed upon the physical object of concentration. The mind becomes one with the object of concentration.

2 **Vichara (savichara and nirvichara samadhis)**. In *savichara* and *nirvichara* the five subtle elements (*tan-matras*) and the subtle senses are the objects of concentration and contemplation. In *savichara* there is concentration on the subtle, aspects of the physical object with reference to space, time and causation. In *nirvichara* the subtle aspects of the object of concentration are not delimited by space, time or causation.

3 *Sananda samadhi* **(ecstasy)**. In *sananda samadhi*, the third *samadhi*, concentration on objects, both gross and subtle, ceases. The intellect becomes quiet, there is no reasoning or reflection. The mind is absorbed in its own inner joy, experiencing the feeling of 'I am joyful', or 'I am blissful'. When this stage of divine bliss has been attained, it is not lost in the further stages of *samadhi*.

4 *Sasmita samadhi*. In *sasmita samadhi*, the fourth *samadhi*, there is only self-awareness (awareness of the 'I'-existence). The self dwells in the Self. The Self is devoid of ego; only the purity of *sattva* dominates in *sasmita samadhi*.

The Highest Stage of *Samadhi*

In *samprajnata samadhi*, also known as *sa-bija samadhi* or *sabikalpa samadhi* – 'subject to time' (*kalpa*) – some duality of subject and object remains. The meditator is unable to remain with his or her consciousness absorbed into the infinite, once he or she comes out of this state. In this *samadhi* the consciousness (*citta*) is still dependent upon an object, symbol or idea for its contemplation.

When through further efforts of deep meditation and absorption in *samadhi*, one reaches the highest stage of *nirbikalpa samadhi* (also known as *nir-bija samadhi*, *asamprajnata samadhi* and *dharma–megha samadhi*). *Nirbikalpa* means 'timeless', it is not subject to change. This is the highest stage of *samadhi*. In this divine state the yogi loses all external consciousness, all awareness of duality and he or she loses the sense of 'I' (*asmita*). The mind, intellect and senses cease to function entirely, and time and space are transcended. There is total absorption.

The yogi who is perfectly established in the perfect awareness of *nirbikalpa samadhi* burns all the residues of his or her actions (*samskaras*). He or she becomes a liberated soul, a *jivanmukta* ('freed while living'). Attaining this exalted state, one does not fall into delusion again.

> *The yogi who has achieved* samadhi *in this life attains liberation, his store of karmas are immediately burnt in the fire of yoga.*
>
> *Vishnu-Purana* 6:7:35

One who has attained *nirbikalpa samadhi* – 'union with god', the summit of spiritual experience – and returns to body-consciousness, continues to function normally in the world, while always remaining in union with the infinite. The enlightened being lives, moves and has his or her being in God at all times.

There are very few souls indeed who attain *nirbikalpa samadhi*, but those yogis who do find the experience to be beyond the realm of thought and words to describe it. If you have never tasted a strawberry before, how can you possibly know exactly what it tastes like by someone describing the taste to you? It is not within your experience, and so it is with *samadhi* – it has to be experienced to know exactly what it is.

Paramhansa Yogananda describes his experience in cosmic consciousness in chapter 14 of his *Autobiography of a Yogi*.

My body became immovably rooted; breath was drawn out of my lungs as if by some huge magnet. Soul and mind instantly lost their physical bondage, and streamed out like a fluid piercing light from my every pore. The flesh was as though dead, yet in my intense awareness I knew that never before had I been fully alive. My sense of identity was no longer narrowly confined to a body, but embraced the circumambient atoms. People on distant streets seemed to be moving gently over my own remote periphery. The roots of plants and trees appeared through a dim transparency of the soil; I discerned the inward flow of their sap...

All objects within my panoramic gaze trembled and vibrated like quick motion pictures. My body, Master's, the pillared courtyard, the furniture and floor, the trees and sunshine, occasionally became violently agitated, until all melted into a luminescent sea; even as sugar crystals, thrown into a glass of water dissolve after being shaken. The unifying light alternated with materializations of form, the metamorphoses revealing the law of cause and effect in creation.

An oceanic joy broke upon calm endless shores of my soul. The Spirit of God, I realized, is exhaustless Bliss; His body is countless tissues of light. A swelling glory within me began to envelop towns, continents, the earth, solar and stellar systems, tenuous nebulae, and floating universes. The entire cosmos, gently luminous, like a city seen afar at night, glimmered within the infinitude of my being. The sharply etched global outlines faded somewhat at the farthest edges; there I could see a mellow radiance, ever-undiminished. It was indescribably subtle; the planetary pictures were formed of a grosser light.

The divine dispersion of rays poured from an Eternal Source, blazing into galaxies, transfigured with ineffable auras. Again and again I saw the creative beams condense into constellations, then resolve into sheets of transparent flame. By rhythmic reversion, sextillion worlds passed into diaphanous lustre; fire became firmament.

I cognized the center of the empyrean as a point of intuitive perception in my heart. Irradiating splendour issued from my nucleus to every part of the universal structure. Blissful amrita, the nectar of immortality, pulsed through me with a quicksilver fluidity. The creative voice of God I heard resounding as aum, the vibration of the Cosmic Motor.

Suddenly the breath returned to my lungs. With a disappointment almost unbearable, I realized that my infinite immensity was lost. Once more I was limited to the humiliating cage of a body, not easily accommodative to the Spirit. Like a prodigal child, I had run away from my macrocosmic home and imprisoned myself in a narrow microcosm.

My guru (Sri Yukteswar) was standing motionless before me; I started to drop at his holy feet in gratitude for the experience in Cosmic Consciousness which I had passionately sought. He held me upright, and spoke calmly, unpretentiously.

'You must not get overdrunk with ecstasy. Much work yet remains for you in the world. Come; let us sweep the balcony floor; then we shall walk by the Ganges.'

FURTHER READING

Arya, Pandit Usharbudhi (known as Swami Veda Bharati), *The Yoga Sutras of Patanjali, with the Exposition of Vyasa, Volume 1, Samadhi Pada*, The Himalayan International Institute of Yoga Science and Philosophy of the USA, Homesdale, Pennsylvania, 1986. *Volume 2, Sadhana Pada*, Motilal Publishers, Dehli, India, 2001

Bhagavad Gita, translated by Eknath Easwaran, Arkana Paperbacks, London, 1986

Desikachar, T K V, *The Heart of Yoga: Developing a Personal Practice*, Inner Traditions International, Rochester, Vermont, 1995

Frawley, Dr David and Dr Subhash Ranade, *Ayurveda – Nature's Medicine*, Lotus Press, Twin Lakes, Wisconsin, 2001

Hatha Yoga Pradipika, commentary by Swami Muktibodhananda Saraswati, Bihar School of Yoga, Ganga Darsha, Munger, Bihar, India, 1993

Kriyananda, Swami, *The Essence of Self-realization: The Wisdom of Paramhansa Yogananda's Words, Preserved and Recorded by his Disciple*, Crystal Clarity Publishers, Nevada City, California, 1990

Mohan, A G, *Yoga for Body, Breath and Mind*, Rudra Press, Cambridge, Massachusetts, 1993

Novak, John (Jyotish), *How to Meditate*, Crystal Clarity Publishers, Nevada City, California, 1989

Rama, Swami, *Living with the Himalayan Masters*, The Himalayan International Institute of Yoga Science and Philosophy of the USA, Homesdale, Pennsylvania

Sargeant, Winthrop, *The Bhagavad Gita*, State University of New York Press, Albany, 1994

Upanishads, translated by Eknath Easwaran, Arkana Paperbacks, London, 1987

Vishudevananda, Swami, *The Complete Illustrated Book of Yoga*, Pocket Books, New York, 1960

FURTHER READING

Walters, J Donald (Swami Kriyananda), *Rays of the Same Light. Parallel Passages with Commentary from the Bible and the Bhagavad Gita* (3 volumes), Crystal Clarity Publishers, Nevada City, California, 1987, 1988, 1989

Walters, J Donald (Swami Kriyananda), *The Path: A Spiritual Autobiography*, Crystal Clarity Publishers, Nevada City, California, 1996

Walters, J Donald (Swami Kriyanada), *Superconsciousness: A Guide to Meditation*, Warner Books, New York, 1996

Ashram-Yogaville, Satchidananda, *The Yoga Sutras of Patanjali*, translation and commentary by Sri Swami Satchidananda, Integral Yoga Publications, Buckingham, Virginia, 1990

Yogananda, Paramhansa, *Autobiography of a Yogi*, Crystal Clarity Publishers, Nevada City, California, reprint of 1946 first edition.

Yogananda, Paramhansa, *Autobiography of a Yogi*, read by Ben Kingsley (audio book edition. 12 audio cassette tapes slipcased). Self-Realization Fellowship, Los Angeles, 1996

Yogananda, Paramhansa, *The Divine Romance*, Self-Realization Fellowship, Los Angeles, California, 1986

Yogananda, Paramhansa, *God Talks with Arjuna: The Bhagavad Gita, Royal Science of God-realization*, Self-Realization Fellowship, Los Angeles, California, 1995

Yogananda, Paramhansa, *In the Sanctuary of the Soul – A Guide to Effective Prayer*, Self-Realization Fellowship, Los Angeles, California, 1998

Yogananda, Paramhansa, *Inner Peace*, Self-Realization Fellowship, Los Angeles, California, 1996

Yogananda, Paramhansa, *Man's Eternal Quest*, Self-Realization Fellowship, Los Angeles, 1975

Yogananda, Paramhansa, *The Rubaiyat of Omar Khayyam Explained*, edited by J Donald Walters (Swami Kriyananda), Crystal Clarity Publishers, Nevada City, California, 1994

Yogananda, Paramhansa, *The Science of Religion*, 3rd edition, Self-Realization Fellowship, Los Angeles, California, 1994

Yogananda, Paramhansa, *Where there is Light, Insights and Inspiration for Meeting Life's Challenges*, Self-Realization Fellowship, Los Angeles, 1988

Yogananda, Paramhansa, *Wine of the Mystic: The Rubaiyat of Omar Khayyam*, Self-Realization Fellowship, Los Angeles, 1994

Yukteswar, Swami Sri, *The Holy Science*, Self-Realization Fellowship, Los Angeles, 1977

USEFUL ADDRESSES

INTERNATIONAL

THE ANANDA CHURCH OF SELF-REALIZATION

Ananda was founded in California in 1967 by Sri Kriyananda, a close direct disciple of the great Master, Paramhansa Yogananda.

The Ananda World Brotherhood Village and The Expanding Light, Ananda's guest retreat, are located near Nevada City, California, in the scenic foothills of the Sierra Nevada Mountains. Ananda Village today has over 350 residents, as well as branch communities in Sacramento, Palo Alto, Portland, Seattle, Dallas and Assisi, Italy. Ananda also supports numerous affiliated meditation groups throughout the world.

The Expanding Light, Ananda's guest retreat, has been a spiritual haven for people from around the world, and from every spiritual background. Here you can experience a holiday retreat that offers a lasting sense of rest and renewal. Here you will have time to step out of your normal routine and gain a fresh new perspective on life, with an opportunity to deepen or begin your spiritual perspectives. This takes place within a friendly, supportive environment that makes it safe for you to open your heart. It is a place for spiritual awakening.

USEFUL ADDRESSES 277

For more details write to:

Ananda Church of Self-Realization
The Expanding Light
14618 Tyler Foote Road
Nevada City
CA 95959, USA
Tel: (800) 346-5350
email: ananda@ananda.org
        info@expandinglight.org
web: www.ananda.org
        www.expandinglight.org

Ananda Church of Self-Realization, founded in 1968 by Kriyananda, a direct disciple of Paramhansa Yogananda, is not affiliated with Self-Realization Fellowship.

AUSTRALIA

There is a new Ananda Centre starting in Brisbane, Australia. For Ananda Meditation groups in Australia contact:

Gayle Marcussen	Ananda Australia
1131 South Pine Road	Karuna & Shoshona McDivitt
Aran Hills	Rodric & Jinnae Anderson
4054 Brisbane	99–107 Main Creek Road
Queensland	Tanawha, Queensland 4556 Australia

EUROPE

The European centre of Ananda was established in Como, northern Italy, in 1984 and transferred to Assisi in 1986. Fifty-five full-time residents from various countries live and work together, creating an atmosphere of loving, joyful co-operation and deep inner peace.

A visit at Ananda is a 'full immersion' in spirituality as a way of life. Classes, meditation, times of silence, vegetarian meals and simple accommodation enable you to live within the context of a spiritual community.

Ananda Assisi is situated in the peaceful hills of Umbria about 10 miles from Assisi, where St Francis lived.

For more details write to:

Ananda Assisi
Casella Postale 48
1-06088 S Maria Degli Angeli (PG)
Italy
Tel: 0742 813620
email: info@ananda.it
web: www.ananda.it

For Ananda meditation groups in the United Kingdom contact:
Stephen Sturgess
52 Nimrod Road
Streatham
London
SW16 6TG
Tel: 0208 696 9832

Richard Fish
Poplar Herb Farm
Burtle
Nr Bridgwater
Somerset
TA7 8NB
Tel: 01278 723170

Please contact Stephen at the above address if you would like him to give day and weekend yoga workshops – Kriya yoga, *pranayama*, meditation, Patanjali's Eight Limbs of Yoga, Mantra chanting.

USA

The Self-Realization Fellowship
3880 San Rafael Avenue
Los Angeles
CA 90065, USA

The Self-Realization Fellowship teach the Science of Kriya Yoga. A comprehensive home-study course, compiled from the writings and lectures of Paramhansa Yogananda. These lessons include step-by-step Kriya Yoga techniques for recharging the body, awakening the power of the mind and expanding the consciousness.

Inspirational videos and tapes and books available. For more information, please request the free booklet, 'Undreamed of Possibilities'.

OTHER RESOURCES

VIDEO TAPES

ANANDA COURSE IN SELF-REALISATION

The *Ananda Course in Self-Realisation* is a complete, practical training programme in yoga, meditation, and the fundamentals of the spiritual path, put together by Swami Sri Kriyananda.

The complete course includes four separate and sequential instructional sections, each in their own ring binder, and 13 audio cassette tapes. In addition, there are a variety of optional supplemental materials, including videos, books and audio cassettes.

KRIYA YOGA AND THE ESSENCE OF YOGA

This fascinating talk offers a complete picture of yoga, from *The Yoga Sutras of Patanjali* to the practice of Raja Yoga.

A COURSE IN MEDITATION – SWAMI SRI KRIYANANDA

This classic approach to meditation is based on the teachings of Paramhansa Yogananda, and on the ancient science of Raja Yoga. In eight half-hour segments, Kriyananda talks in depth about the fundamental techniques of concentration, how to receive inner guidance, and the eight aspects of God that serve as the basis for deeper meditation. Taught with warmth and spiritual power.

LESSONS IN YOGA: 14 STEPS TO HIGHER AWARENESS – SWAMI SRI KRIYANANDA

A seven-month home study correspondence course which is a multidimensional approach to yoga and meditation. Each of the 14 lessons includes sections on yoga philosophy, yoga postures, breathing, daily yoga routine, diet, healing and meditation. The course includes 14 printed lessons mailed bi-weekly and 16 cassette tapes of original companion talks by Kriyananda.

Both the above are available from:

Ananda Church of Self-Realisation
14618 Tyler Foot Rd
Nevada City
CA 95959
Tel: (916) 478-7560

AUDIO TAPES

Inspiring talks on yoga, meditation, *The Yoga Sutras of Patanjali* and other related subjects on spirituality by Swami Veda Bharati (formally Pandit Usharbudh Arya) who is a disciple of Swami Rama of the Himalayan Institute of Yoga and Philosophical Studies.

Swami Veda Bharati is the founder and director of the meditation centre in Minneapolis, an affiliate of the Himalayan Institute of Yoga Sciences and Philosophy. He has recorded 5,000 hours of tapes.

If you are interested in studying *The Yoga Sutras of Patanjali* then I recommend you write for a list of his tapes to the following address:

The Meditation Centre
631 University Avenue NE
Minneapolis
Minnesota 55413
USA
Tel: (612) 379 2386

Glossary

ABHYANTARA KUMBHAKA Internal breath retention.

ABHYASA Constant and determined spiritual practice.

ADHAM PRANAYAMA Abdominal breathing.

ADHIBHAUTIKA Pain caused by other beings (including wild animals and insects).

ADHIDAIVIKA Pain or suffering caused by natural forces (by sound, air, fire, water, earth or by planetary forces).

ADHYAM PRANAYAMA Upper or clavicular breathing.

ADHYATMIKA Pain within oneself (physical, mental and emotional).

AGAMI KARMAS The actions which are being done in this present life and will bear fruits in a future life.

AGNI SARA DHAUTI Fire purification (purifies the *nadis*).

AHAM 'I am'.

AHAMKARA Ego; identifying faculty.

AHAT NADA All external or 'struck' sounds such as musical instruments played.

AHIMSA Non-violence, non-injury, non-harming.

AJAPA-JAPA The spontaneous and automatic repetition of a mantra, without conscious effort.

ALABDHA BHUMIKATVA Unsuccessful in gaining a firm ground in yoga.

ALAMBANA Objective support; dependent on.

ALASYA Sloth; lethargy.

AMRITA Nectar.

ANAHATA CHAKRA The centre of consciousness at the heart.

ANAHATA NADA All sounds which do not have any external source or 'unstruck' sound.

ANANDA Joy, bliss.

ANANDA-SANANDA SAMADHI In this *samadhi* concentration on objects, both gross and subtle, ceases. The mind is absorbed in its own inner joy; ecstasy.

Glossary

ANANDAMAYA KOSHA The bliss sheath. It is the cause of both the subtle and gross bodies.

ANAVASTHITATTVA Instability; unsteadiness of mind.

ANGA A limb or part of the body.

ANNAMAYA KOSHA The food sheath. The physical sheath of the gross body.

ANTAHKARANA Literally means 'inner instrument'; inner organ of consciousness.

ANTAR Inner, internal.

ANTAR DHAUTI Internal washing of the digestive tract.

ANULOMA-VILOMA Classical *pranayama*; Alternate nostril breathing; purifies the subtle nerves and calms the mind.

APANA One of the five major *vayus*; functions in the region of the navel to the feet.

APARIGRAHA Non-attachment; non-greed.

ARDHA-PADMASANA Half-lotus pose.

ASAMPRAJNATA SAMADHI Also known as *nir-bija samadhi*, 'without support' or 'seedless' and *nirodha samadhi* – total control and final cessation of mental fluctuations (*vrittis*).

ASANA posture; A posture that brings steadiness to the body and calmness to the mind.

ASHTANGA YOGA (*ashta* 'eight'; *anga* 'limb') The eight-fold path. The system described by the sage, Patanjali in the *Yoga Sutras*.

ASHWINI MUDRA Horse *mudra*; contraction of the anal sphincter muscles.

ASMITA I-am-ness; the sense of 'I'.

ASTA Eight.

ASTEYA Non-stealing.

ATMA Self, the eternal, individual soul.

ATMAN Self, soul.

AUM The sacred primordial sound '*om*' is the root of all mantras; the orgin of all sounds and contains all sounds; emanating from the Holy Ghost.

AUM-TAT-SAT *Aum*, the creative sound vibration word-symbol for God; *Tat*.the cosmic intelligence of spirit or the Christ consciousness, *Sat*, truth.

AVATAR (literally, 'one who descends') A plenary or partial incaranation of God who appears in the world to carry out a particular divine mission.

AVIRATI Attachment to sense-pleasure.

BAHYA KUMBHAKA External breath retention.

BAHYA-VISAYA External object.

BANDHA Lock.

BASTI Colon cleansing (water enema).

BHADRASANA Nobility pose.

BHAGAVAD GITA 'The Song of the Lord', name of a scripture consisting of 18 chapters from the *Mahabharata* epic. It is a dialogue between Lord Krishna and his disciple Arjuna.

BHAKTI YOGA (*bhaj* to serve, love, worship) The path of love and devotion.

BHASTRIKA PRANAYAMA Bellows breath. Like a bellows used by a blacksmith in a furnace, where the air is forcibly drawn in and out.

BHRAMARI Humming Bee breath; produces the sound of a bee.

BHRANTI-DARSHANA Distorted vision; philosophical confusion; delusion.

BIJA Seed.

BIJA MANTRA A mystical seed-syllable sound.

BRAHMA God the creator.

BRAHMACHARYA Purity, non-sensuality.

BRAHMA-SUTRAS Ancient Vedic scriptures.

BRAHMAMUHURTA 'The hour of God'. The auspicious hours of meditation, between 4.00 am and 6.00 am.

BRIHADARANYAKA UPANISHAD Vedic scripture, which is the oldest of the Upanishads (800 BC).

BUDDHI Intellect; discriminating faculty.

CHACKSHU DHAUTI Cleaning the eyes.

CHAKRAS ('wheels') The seven subtle centres of consciousness, situated in the subtle spine (*sushumna*) in the astral body; Revolving vortices of energy.

CHANDRA Moon.

CIT Pure consciousness.

CITTA Field of consciousness (mind-intellect-ego).

DANTA DHAUTI Cleaning the teeth.

DEVADATHA Minor *prana*: controls yawning.

DEVAS Gods.

DHANANJAYA Minor *prana*: controls the decomposition of the body after death.

DHANURASANA The bow pose.

DHARANA Concentration of the mind's attention to one particular point. From the word dhri ('to hold firm').

DHARMA-MEGHA SAMADHI The final state of *samprajnata samadhi*; *dharma* means 'virtue' and *megha* means 'rain cloud'. The *samadhi* of the rain cloud of virtue.

DHATU One of the seven basic tissues of the body.

DHYANA Meditation.

GLOSSARY 285

DOHANA Milking the tongue.

DOSHAS The three basic types of biological energy which determine individual constitution: vata, pitta and kapha.

DUHKHA Pain, grief and sorrow.

DVESHA Disapproval.

EKA One.

EKAGRATA (One-pointed) attention.

GHERANDA SAMHITA One of the main ancient texts on Hatha Yoga by Yogi Gheranda.

GOMUKHASANA Cow's-head pose.

GORAKSHA SAMHITA Classical treatise on Hatha Yoga by Yogi Gorakhnath (11th century).

GRANTHI Knot.

GUNA Qualities of nature: *sattva*, *rajas* and *tamas*.

GURU Spiritual Master.

HALASANA Plough pose.

HATHA Hatha consists of two letters: *Ha* (sun) and *tha* (moon).

HATHA YOGA A system of purifying techniques and yoga postures to control the mind through control of *prana*. Hatha Yoga prepares the student for Raja Yoga. It promotes good health, giving control over the body and mind.

HATHA YOGA PRADIPIKA 15th-century treatise on the practice of Hatha Yoga by Svatmarama

HONG SAU Kriya mantra for developing deep concentration ('I am He').

HRID DHAUTI Cleaning the throat.

IDA One of the main *nadis* (subtle nerve channels) on the left side of *sushumna*; associated with cool moon.

ISVARAPRANIDHANA Surrender of oneself to God.

JAGRAT Waking state of consciousness.

JALANDHARA BANDHA Chin lock. *Jala* means 'net' or 'network'. In the neck there is a network of nerves and arteries. Dhara means 'pulling upwards'.

JAPA Repetition; repetition of a mantra.

JIVANMUKTA 'Freed while living'; liberated soul.

JNANA YOGA (*jna* 'to know') The path of wisdom.

KALPA Time.

KANDA Junction of *sushumna* and *muladhara chakra*. From here the *nadis* distribute the *prana* all over the body; a knot.

KAPALABHATI Frontal brain purification (*kapala* means 'skull' and *bhati* means 'shine').

KARIKARA Minor *prana*: controls sneezing and induces hunger and thirst.

KARMA (*kri* 'to do, to act') Action; former actions which will lead to certain results in a cause/effect relationship.

KARMA YOGA The path of selfless action.

KARNA DHAUTI Cleaning the ears.

KATI CHAKRASANA Waist-rotating pose.

KECHARI MUDRA Tongue lock; *Kha* means *akasha* ('space') and *chari* means 'to move', so *kechari mudra* means 'moving-in-space position'.

KEVAL KUMBHAKA Spontaneous suspension of the breath.

KIRTAN Devotional chanting.

KLESHA Pain, suffering.

KLISHTA Painful.

KOSHAS 'sheaths'.

KRIPA Grace.

KRISHNA The eighth incarnation of Lord Vishnu; 'all-attractive'; 'black' or 'the Dark One'. Krishna revealed the teachings of the Bhagavad Gita to Arjuna.

KRIYA YOGA (*kri* 'to do, to act') Union with God through a certain action or rite. Kriya Yoga was revived in this age by the great Himalayan Yogi, Mahavatar Babaji.

KUMBHAK Retention of breath.

KUNDALINI The coiled-up, dormant, cosmic energy. The *kundalini*, which gives power and energy to all the chakras, lies at the *muladhara chakra* (base of spine).

KUNJAL KRIYA Upper digestive tract cleansing.

KURMA minor *prana*: controls the function of opening the eyelids and causes vision.

LAYA Dissolution; absorption of the mind.

LIKHITA JAPA Writing a mantra.

LOMA PRANAYAMA Three-part equal-breath ratio.

MADHYAM PRANAYAMA Middle or intercostal breathing.

MAHA MUDRA The great seal.

MAHA VEDHA MUDRA Great piercing *mudra*.

MAHARSI A great sage.

MAHASAMADHI the final superconscious meditation, in which a perfected Spiritual Master departs consciously from the physical body in Divine union with God.

MALA A garland.

MANAS Mind; recording faculty.

MANASIKA JAPA Repeating a mantra mentally.

MANIPURA CHAKRA The centre of consciousness at the level of the navel.

MANOMAYA KOSHA The mental sheath. It is more subtle than the vital pranic sheath.

MANTRA From *manas* ('mind') and *tri* ('to cross over') Mantra liberates the consciousness, it helps one to cross over the sea of the uncontrolled and conditioned mind.

MANTRAS Sound-syllables that have a spiritual vibratory potency.

MATSYASANA Fish pose.

MAYA Illusion, the power which makes form appear as reality; 'that which is not'.

MULABANDHA Anal lock.

MULADHARA CHAKRA The centre of consciousness at the base of the spine, where *kundalini* resides.

MURCHA PRANAYAMA The fainting *pranayama*, induces calm and tranquillity to the mind.

NABHO MUDRA Sky *mudra*.

NADA Inner sound.

NADI SHUDDHI Subtle nerve purifying *pranayama*. This *pranayama* is also known as *anuloma-viloma* when the addition of breath retention is used.

NADIS Subtle nerve channels, through which energy flows in the subtle body.

NAGA Minor *prana*: controls the function of belching and hiccoughing; gives rise to consciousness.

NAGA PRANAYAMA A *pranayama* for purifying the skin.

NARADA SUTRAS The philosophy of love and devotion by the ancient holy sage, Narada.

NAULI Abdominal massage; contracting and isolating the rectus abdominal muscles.

NAULI KRIYA Intestinal wash.

NETI Nasal cleansing.

NIDRA Sleep; *yoga nidra* means 'psychic sleep of the yogis'.

NIRALAMBANA No objective support in meditation.

NIRBIKALPA SAMADHI Timeless *samadhi*, it is not subject to change. This is the highest stage of *samadhi*.

NIRGUNA Formless.

NIRVICHARA SAMADHI *Samadhi* without subtle thought.

NIRVIKALPA SAMADHI *Samadhi* in which the duality of subject and object is completely transcended.

NIRVITARKA SAMADHI *Samadhi* without a gross thought.

NIRVITARKA SAMAPATTI At this stage of *samadhi* there is no word-object-idea from memory superimposed upon the physical object of concentration.

NIYAMA Five individual ethical observances of yoga.

OJAS Vitality, energy.

PADADIRASANA Breath-balancing pose.

PADANGUSTHASANA Toe-balance pose.

PADMASANA Lotus pose.

PARAMHANSA 'Supreme Swan'; *Param* means 'great' or 'supreme'. *Hansa* means 'swan'. Symbolizes spiritual discrimination.

PATANJALI The ancient illumined author of the *Yoga Sutras*.

PINGALA One of the main *nadis* (subtle nerve channels) on the right side of the *sushumna*; associated with heat; sun.

PRAKRITI Supreme Matter; nature.

PRAMADA Carelessness; negligence.

PRANA Life-force, vital energy.

PRANAMAYA KOSHA The vital or etheric sheath; pranic body.

PRANAVA The sacred syllable *aum* (*om*).

PRANAYAMA Control of the life-energy through the breath.

PRARABDHA KARMAS The actions which have given the present life and have already started to bear fruit.

PRATYAHARA Interiorization of the mind, by reversing the senses' outward attention from external objects, to their source within.

PURAK Inhalation.

PURANAS Ancient Vedic scriptures that contain hundreds of thousands of verses.

PURUSHA Supreme Spirit.

RAGA Approval.

RAJA YOGA (*raja* 'royal') The royal path; the yoga path of meditation.

RAJASIC (RAJAS) The mode of passion and desire.

RAMANA MAHARSHI A great spiritual teacher of India (1879–1950). At the age of 17 he attained a profound experience of the true Self without the guidance of a guru.

RECHAK Exhalation.

RUDRA Shiva as Destroyer.

SABIKALPA SAMADHI 'Subject to time'; In this *samadhi*, some duality of subject and object remains.

SADHANA Path of spiritual discipline.

SAGUNA With form.

Glossary

SAH He (the universal Spirit).

SAHASRARA The centre of consciousness located at the top of the head. The crown chakra; the thousand-petalled lotus.

SAMADHI Superconsciousness; absorption. Samadhi is attained when the meditator, the process of meditation and the object of meditation become one. Union with God.

SAMADHI Superconsciousness; absorption.

SAMANA One of the five major *vayus*; functions between the heart and navel.

SAMAPATTI Attainment of a state of consciousness.

SAMATA Equanimity, or equal-mindedness.

SAMITA SAMADHI In this *samadhi* the self is devoid of ego. The self dwells in the self.

SAMPATTI Perfection; fulfilment.

SAMPRAJNATA SAMADHI Lower *samadhi* also known as *sa-bija samadhi*, 'with support' or 'with seed'. The *samadhi* of wisdom.

SAMSHAYA Doubt.

SAMSKARAS Deep mental impressions produced by past experiences; dormant impressions of our past lives.

SANCHITA KARMAS The actions that have accumulated in several previous lifetimes.

SANTOSHA Contentment.

SARVANGASANA Shoulder stand.

SAT Being, pure Truth.

SATCIDANANDA Pure being – pure consciousness – absolute bliss.

SATSANGA Association with spiritually orientated people.

SATTVIC (SATTVA) The mode of goodness, purity – the highest of the three gunas.

SATYA Truth, truthfulness.

SAUCHA Cleanliness, purity.

SAVICHARA SAMADHI *Samadhi* with subtle thought.

SAVIKALPA SAMADHI *Samadhi* in which some duality of subject and object remains.

SAVITARKA SAMADHI The lowest *samadhi*; *samadhi* with gross thought.

SAVITRE PRANAYAMA The difference between *savitre* and *savitri pranayamas* is that the breathing ratio is reversed in savitre.

SAVITRI PRANAYAMA The rhythmic breath; harmonizing; uses a four-part breath ratio.

SHAKTI The power and energy of consciousness.

SHANKHAPRAKSHALANA (also known as *varisara dhauti*) *Shank* meaning 'conch shell', which has convolutions resembling the intestines; *prakshalana* meaning 'to wash thoroughly'. Complete cleansing of the entire digestive and eliminative systems.

SHANTI Perfect peace, tranquillity.

SHAT KRIYAS Internal purification techniques.

SHATKARMAS Cleansing technique.

SHIVA Auspicious, the third deity of the Hindu Trinity, Shiva the Destroyer, who brings about the destruction of the ego.

SHIVA SAMHITA Classical treatise on Hatha Yoga (late 17th century).

SHUNYA Vacuum or void.

SIDDHA Perfected being.

SIDDHA YONI ASANA The female accomplished pose.

SIDDHASANA Perfect pose; adept's pose; accomplished pose.

SIDDHI Psychic power.

SIRSHASANA Headstand.

SITALI A *pranayama* that cools the body system.

SITKARI A *pranayama* that cools the body system.

SMRITI Memory.

SOHAM The natural mantric sound of the breath.

SRIMAD-BHAGAVATAM *Bhagavata Purana*, the most popular of the 18 *Puranas* are scriptures of the *bhakti* (devotion) path.

STYANA Mental laziness; procrastination.

SUKHASANA The easy pose.

SUKSMA SARIRA Subtle body.

SUKYA PRANAYAMA Pleasant breath.

SUMERU Mount Meru.

SURYA BHEDA *Surya* ('sun'); *bheda* ('to pierce'). *Surya bheda pranayama* activates the solar, right nostril.

SUSHUMNA The central channel or *nadi* of the subtle body, which the *kundalini* ascends through.

SUSHUPTI Dreamless sleep.

SUTRA Thread; an aphorism.

SUTRA NETI Nasal cleansing with string.

SVADHISHTHANA CHAKRA The centre of consciousness at the level of the genitals.

SVADHYAYA Self-study.

SWAMI 'Master of the senses', one who is awakened to the self within (*swa*).

SWAPNA Dream state of consciousness.

SWARA YOGA The science of the flow of *prana*.

SWASTIKASANA The auspicious pose.

TAMASIC (TAMAS) The mode of ignorance, inertia – the lowest of the three gunas.

TANTRIC YOGA Expression of consciousness; a spiritual path that expands the consciousness using mantras, ritual, meditation, workshop of the Goddess and her Lord Shiva. Tantra's basic principle is *shakti* (female power).

TAPAS Austerity; heat; inner fire.

TATTVA Elements; five states of energy matter (ether, air, fire, water, earth).

TIRYAKA BHUJANGASANA Twisting cobra pose.

TRATAK Gazing with concentration at an object.

TRI Three.

TRIDOSHA The three *doshas* – *vata* (air/ether), *pitta* (fire/water), *kapha* (water/earth). Govern all the functions of the body, mind and consciousness.

UDANA One of the five major *vayus*; functions in the body above the larynx and the top of the head.

UDARAKARSHANASANA Stomach-squeezing pose.

UDDIYANA BANDHA Abdominal lock.

UJJAYI PRANAYAMA The Sanskrit prefix *ud* means 'to raise upwards'. *Jaya* means 'victorious'. *Pranayama* in which the glottis of the throat is slightly contracted to produce continuous hissing sound.

UPANISHAD A division of Vedic literature, consisting of 108 metaphysical texts.

UPANSU JAPA Whispering a mantra.

VAIKHARI JAPA Speaking or chanting a mantra aloud.

VAIRAGYA Detachment; freedom from wordly desires; dispassion.

VAJRA NADI Psychic channel.

VAJRASANA Thunderbolt pose.

VAJROLI MUDRA The thunderbolt *mudra*.

VAMANA DHAUTI Upper digestive tract cleansing.

VASTRA DHAUTI Internal cleansing of digestive tract using a strip of finely woven muslin cloth, one metre long.

VAYU Air.

VIBHAGA PRANAYAMA Sectional breathing.

VIBHUTI PADA Third part of *The Yoga Sutras of Patanjali* which goes into the properties of yoga and the art of integration through concentration, meditation and *samadhi*.

VICHARA Subtle thought; contemplation.

VIJNANAMAYA KOSHA The intelligent sheath.

VIKALPA Imagination.

VILOMA PRANAYAMA Inverse breathing.

VIPAREET KARANI MUDRA Reverse posture *mudra*.

VIRYASTAMBHANASANA Semen-retention pose.

VISHNU 'The all-pervading one'. 'The Preserver'; Vishnu descends to earth in the form of a divine incarnation, such as Krishna and Buddha.

VISHNU MUDRA Hand *mudra* used in alternate nostril breathing.

VISHUDDHI CHAKRA The centre of consciousness at the level of the throat.

VITARKA Gross thought.

VRITTIS Thought waves; modifications of the mind-field.

VYADHI Disease.

VYANA One of the five major *vayus*; functions throughout the whole body.

YAMA Five ethical disciplines of yoga.

YOGA (*yuj* 'to unite') spiritual union; a path to Self-realization.

YOGA MUDRA Yogic seal.

YOGANANDA PARAMHANSA A great spiritual Master (avatar) born in India, 1893. He left his body in *mahasamadhi* in 1952. Yogananda brought Kriya Yoga to the West.

YOGI One who practises yoga.

YONI MUDRA *Yoni* means 'the womb' and *mudra* means 'seal'.

INDEX

abdominal breathing 194, 195–6, 200
abdominal muscles 119, 123, 130, 131, 138–9, 260
abdominal organs 156, 159, 162, 164
adham pranayama (*see* abdominal breathing)
adhi mudra 201, 202
adhyam pranayama (*see* clavicular breathing)
adrenal glands 156
affirmation 28–9
agni sara dhauti 117, 119–20 146, 190
ahimsa 24, 25, 26–30
air 9, 10, 92, 193, 219
ajapa japa 81–3
ajna chakra (*see* spiritual eye)
akasha (*see* ether)
alabdha bhumikatva (*see* failure to progress)
alasya (*see* laziness)
alcohol 52–3, 57, 75, 220
allergies 125
anahata chakra 10, 15–16, 22, 183, 237, 238
Ananda Church of God-realization 258, 266
anandamaya kosha 5
anasthitatva (*see* instability)
annamaya kosha 1, 5, 13

Anthony, St 62
anuloma-viloma pranayama (see *nadi shuddhi*)
anxiety 136, 144, 210
apana vayu 4, 123, 154, 157, 177, 207, 210
aparigraha 25, 46–8
ardha padmasana 251–2
asamprajnata samadhi (*nirbikalpa samadhi*) 12, 270, 272
asana (postures) 12, 24, 27, 55, 78, 110–12, 114, 135, 145, 147, 150, 169, 178, 186, 189, 190, 218, 219, 230, 233, 258
(*see also* individual *asanas*)
asceticism 62–3, 64
Ashtanga Yoga 23–4
ashwini mudra 43, 146, 157, 159–60, 190
asteya 24, 25, 32–5
asthma 119, 125, 210, 259
astral body 1, 5, 6, 8, 10, 20, 57, 164, 172, 176, 189
Atman (*see* Self)
attachment 45, 46, 48, 60, 61, 64, 75, 109, 221
attraction 174, 175
aum 83–6, 265, 266
aum-tat-sat 84
austerity (see *tapas*)
autonomic nervous system 143, 161, 177

aversion 174, 175
avidya (see ignorance)
avirati (see attachment)
awareness 68–70, 71, 74, 76, 90, 210, 221, 228, 261
Ayurveda 117

Baba, Devraha 186
Baba, Shivapuri 186
Babaji, Mahavatar 35, 186, 250, 262–3, 264, 265
Bacon, Francis 70
bandhas 43, 114, 154, 158, 192, 193, 249 (see also individual bandhas)
bhadrasana 43, 112
Bhagavad Gita 7, 38, 45, 48, 59, 63–5, 67, 75, 76, 86, 92, 98, 99–100, 103, 105, 107, 109, 149, 152, 153, 222–3, 257, 263
Bhakti Yoga 114
bhastrika pranayama 137, 143, 144, 178, 204–7, 226
bhramari pranayama 211
bhranti darshana (see distorted vision)
bhujangasana 258, 259
Bible 45, 84, 97, 98, 109
bile 117, 119
bliss sheath (see anandamaya kosha)
blood 123, 139, 142, 181, 199, 205, 210, 227
body 37, 51–2, 62, 63, 64, 65, 69, 70–1, 90, 94, 110, 113, 147, 219, 240 (see also astral, causal and physical bodies)
bowel 123
Brahma 84, 102
Brahmachari, Lokanath 186
brahmacharya 24, 25, 35–46, 51
brahma mudra 200, 201–2
brahmamuhurta 243, 255
Brahman (see supreme Reality)

Brahma-Sutras 98
Brahma-Vaivarta Purana 148
breath 81–2, 86, 169–70, 172, 180–2, 184–6, 187–9, 200, 225, 230, 233, 243, 261
breath retention 157, 158, 169, 170, 183, 191, 192, 205, 207, 209
Brihadaranyaka Upanishad 189
Buddha 27, 101, 148

carelessness (see negligence)
catarrh 136
causal body 1, 5, 6
central nervous system 143
chakras 8–10, 12–22, 81–2, 161, 183 (see also individual chakras)
chakrasana 129, 131, 179
chalana 167
chandra bhedana 179
chandra bheda pranayama 208
chanting (see japa)
chinmaya mudra 200, 201, 202
chin mudra 200, 201, 202, 249
chitta (see subconscious)
Christ-consciousness 18, 84
clavicular breathing 194–5, 197, 200–1
coffee 52, 54
colds 136
colon 124
consciousness 9, 12, 17, 31, 51, 56, 60, 67, 68, 70, 72, 79, 89, 90, 104, 147, 168, 172, 224–5, 228, 232, 240, 264, 272
constipation 119, 120, 125, 139, 156, 158, 160, 163, 164
contentment (see santosha)
cosmic Consciousness 17, 33, 83, 236, 264, 273
coughs 136
crown chakra (see sahasrara chakra)
curiosity 219

dakshina nauli 124, 142
danta dhauti 117, 120–2, 150
death 6–8, 171, 174, 175, 176
depression 136, 144, 210
desire 32–3, 37, 45, 59, 60, 75, 109, 221
despair 77–8
devadatha 177
dhananjaya 177
dhanurasana 129, 130, 259, 260
dharana (concentration) 24, 111, 213, 218, 224, 228–33, 239, 269 (*see also* individual concentration techniques)
dharma-megha samadhi (see *samprajnata samadhi*)
dhauti 112, 117–22
dhyana (*see* meditation)
diabetes 130, 260
diaphragm 156
diaphragmatic breathing (*see* abdominal breathing)
diet 52–3, 146–7, 151–2, 254
digestive organs 137, 204
digestive problems 118, 123, 125, 156, 162, 180, 210
disease 70–1, 93, 216
distorted vision 76
divine Consciousness (*see* cosmic Consciousness)
divine union (see *samadhi*)
dohana 167
doubt 74
dreamless sleep (see *sushupti*)
dream state (see *swapna*)
drugs 52, 53, 57, 75, 220
dukha (*see* pain)
dyspepsia 119, 139, 164

ears 122
earth 3, 8, 10, 13, 92, 193, 219
ego 5, 7, 14, 17, 28, 31, 32, 36, 37–8, 60, 68, 74, 75, 89, 90–2, 107, 109, 148, 173, 174, 175, 220–1, 228, 230, 232, 240–1, 261, 269, 271
egotism 27, 62, 64, 89, 91
Ekadasi 148, 149
elimination organs 204
emotions 225
endocrine glands 19–20, 139, 210
energization exercises 171, 258, 265, 266
energy 9, 10, 17, 18, 20, 31, 39, 62, 73, 113, 148, 158, 173, 234, 243, 258
environment 57
equanimity 59
ether (*akasha*) 3, 9, 10, 16, 92, 165, 219
exhalation 78, 169, 170, 178, 183, 191, 209
eyes 122, 136, 137, 145

failure to progress 76
faith 105–6
fasting 146–52
fear 60, 174, 175, 221
fire 3, 9, 10, 14, 92, 193, 219
food preparation 153
food sheath (see *annamaya kosha*)
forehead 122
Francis, St 27, 93, 101, 148
freedom 63, 94

Gandhi, Mahatma 27
gastric fire 156, 158, 162, 205
gastritis, 119
Gheranda Samhita 111, 143, 158, 184, 208
God 9, 15, 25, 30, 36, 65, 70, 72, 83, 85, 92, 222
 as focus for concentration 231–2
 as infinite 241
 as love 94, 95, 97, 101–2
 as one 102–3
 as security 47, 105

as source of everything 47, 89, 99–100
as Truth 31, 94
communion with 31, 35, 55–6, 93–4
devotion to 106–7, 108, 253, 261
existence of 73–4
formless and with form 101–2
grace of 103–4, 106
law of 96
Name of 79–81, 86, 88, 107, 237, 261
nature of 93–105
offering food to 153–4
our relationship with 33, 45–6, 48–9, 51, 65
surrender to 33, 55, 61, 88–9, 91–3, 104, 108, 109
Will of 34, 48, 61, 65, 73, 74, 95, 99, 108, 109
within us 67–8, 94, 95, 97–8, 100–1, 109, 238, 240, 262
gomukhasana 44
Gorakshanath 112
Goraksha Samhita 112
gorakshasana (see *bhadrasana*)
greed 32–3
gunas 174
Gyanamata, Sister 108

halasana 159, 226–7
hang sah 81
happiness 57, 59
Hatha Yoga 110, 111–15 (see also individual practices)
Hatha Yoga Pradipika 111, 112, 117, 123, 139, 165, 171, 172, 173
hay fever 136
headaches 118
health 113, 147
heart 156, 162, 204, 210, 227
hong sau 81, 82, 234–6, 261, 265, 266

hypertension 210
hysteria 136

'I-am-ness' (see ego)
ida nadi 11, 17, 18, 111, 136, 165, 187–9, 190, 206, 208, 234
ignorance 27, 28, 60, 67, 70, 75, 89–91, 92, 101, 175, 220, 228, 271
imagination 59, 60, 61
inhalation 78, 169, 170, 183, 191, 209
insomnia 144, 210
instability 77
intellect 5, 91, 173, 240–1
intelligent sheath (see *vijnamaya kosha*)
intercostal breathing 194, 196–7, 200
intestines 123, 124, 128, 139
introspection 31, 32, 37, 67, 72–3
Isa-Upanishad 81
isvarapranidhana 50, 89, 108

jagrat 1
jala (see water)
jalandhara bandha 43, 141, 155, 157, 158, 161, 192, 198–9, 204, 205, 206, 207–8, 209, 210, 211, 212, 214
jala neti 117, 131, 136–7, 138, 143, 179
japa (chanting) 66, 79–81, 85, 106, 226, 237
Jaya 267
Jesus Christ 16, 17, 27, 33, 47–8, 56, 67, 76, 84, 93, 101, 106, 148, 236, 241, 242, 263, 264, 265
jnana mudra (see *chinmaya mudra*)
John the Baptist 84
joy 33, 49, 61, 63, 73, 89, 93, 94, 97, 172, 221 223, 232, 262

Jyotish 267

kanda 189
kapalbhati 112, 117, 137, 142–4, 146, 178, 190, 207, 226
karikara 177
karma 6, 13, 18, 59, 96, 270
karnapidasana 226–7
kati chakrasana 128
kechari mudra 164, 165–8, 189
kicheri 131–3
kidneys 119, 125, 139, 150, 227, 259
kirtan 107, 226, 238
kleshas 174–5, 270
koshas 1, 8 (*see also* individual koshas)
Krishna 7, 38, 48, 59, 63–5, 67, 75, 76, 92, 101, 149, 177, 196, 222, 236, 242, 257–8
Kriyananda, Sri 12, 17, 38, 106, 115, 153, 165, 229, 234–5, 265, 266, 267
Kriya Yoga 10, 12, 66, 82, 114, 226, 258, 262–8
kumbhak (*see* breath retention)
kundalini 3, 4, 13, 114–15, 143, 154, 158, 160, 168, 176, 189, 204, 205, 208
Kundalini Yoga 10, 114
kunjal kriya 118, 131
kurma 177
Kurma Purana 230–1

laghoo shankhaprakshalana 134, 149, 150
lam 193
Lawrence, Brother 109
Laya Yoga 10, 114
laziness 75
liver 119, 130, 128, 139, 150, 164, 204, 227, 259, 260
loma pranayama 203, 235, 260
longevity 191–3

love 15, 30, 32, 33, 36, 38, 47, 49, 56, 79, 89, 93, 94, 97, 106–7, 172, 232, 262
low breathing (*see* abdominal breathing)
lungs 119, 162, 180, 181, 184, 199, 200, 203–4, 205

Ma, Sri Anandamayi 93, 105, 241
madhyama nauli 124, 141
madhyam pranayama (*see* intercostal breathing)
mahabandha 43, 158, 161
maha mudra 160–1, 258
Maharshi, Ramana 103
Mahasaya, Lahiri 35, 186, 250, 262–3, 263, 264–5
maha vedha mudra 161
mala beads 86–8, 237
manomaya kosha 4
manipura chakra 10, 14, 22, 120, 156, 157, 162, 164, 183
mantra 79–88, 234
matsyasana 42, 179
Matsyendranath 112
matter 9
meat 52, 54, 75
meditation (*dhyana*) 23, 24, 27, 38, 46, 55–6, 61, 63, 73, 74, 77, 78, 81, 94, 108, 111, 112, 134, 175, 186, 218, 230–1, 233, 239–42, 257–8, 265, 269–70 (*see also* individual meditation postures)
depth 244–5
in a chair 246–7
length 244
place 242–3
technique 258–61
thoughts in 256–7
time 243
waking for 252–6
medulla oblongata 4, 8, 17, 20, 82, 168

memory 59, 60, 61, 162
mental laziness 72–4, 75
middle breathing (see intercostal breathing)
migraines 125
mind 7, 28–9, 37, 51, 57, 62, 63, 67, 173, 219, 232, 240–1
  contentment in 58–61
  control of 45, 65, 69, 148
  healthy 70–1, 113
  inability to understand God 93–4
  interiorization of 228, 233–6, 261
  purity of 55–6, 147
  relationship with senses and soul 90–1, 219–20
  stillness of 31–2, 68, 78, 90, 92, 110, 240
moderation 38, 61, 146
moods 77–8
moon 17, 111, 119, 187–8, 193
mucus 117, 118, 119, 120, 134, 135, 136, 142
mudras 43, 112, 114, 157, 158, 200–1 (see also individual mudras)
Muktananda, Swami 241
mulabandha 43, 154, 158, 160, 161, 182, 205, 206, 208, 209
muladhara chakra 3, 8, 10, 11, 13, 22, 81, 82, 83, 114, 162, 183, 189, 205, 251
murcha pranayama 212

nabho mudra 167
nada 15, 211, 226
Nada Yoga 168
nadis 10–11, 18, 55, 114, 116, 120, 125, 143, 146, 161, 173, 177, 189–90, 193, 204 (see also individual nadis)
nadi shuddhi (anuloma-viloma pranyama) 10, 146, 179, 190–3, 207, 260

naga 177
naga pranayama 214–15
Narada 15
Narada Sutras 107
nauli 112, 117, 123, 139–42, 156, 189
negligence 74
nerve plexuses 8, 20, 140
nerves 143, 144, 159, 177, 204, 227, 259
neti 112, 117, 135–8
nirbija samadhi (see asamprajnata samadhi)
nirbikalpa samadhi (see asamprajnata samadhi)
nirvichara samadhi 271
nirvitarka samadhi 271
niyama 24, 50, 67, 218 (see also individual niyamas)
nose 135, 137, 182

ojas shakti 39
om 17, 22, 81, 83–6, 94, 97, 234, 260, 261

padadirasana 181, 189
padangushthasana 41–2
padmasana 144, 155, 162, 178, 193, 205, 207, 212, 246, 248, 250–1
pain 27, 37, 56, 63, 77, 221
pancha sahita pranayama 203–4
pancreas 119, 130, 139, 227, 260
Parvati 112
pashinee mudra 124, 159
Patanjali 23, 24, 25, 26–7, 50, 58–9, 60, 62, 66, 70, 76, 85, 88, 110, 113, 114, 169–71, 174–6, 218, 228, 229, 239, 269, 270–1
Paul, St 97
pavanamuktasana 129–30
peace 33, 49, 61, 63, 89, 93, 94, 97, 221, 223, 232, 262

INDEX 299

philosophical confusion 75–6
physical body 1–5, 10, 20, 51,
  164, 171, 176, 241
piles 158, 160, 164
pingala nadi 11, 17, 18, 111, 136,
  165, 187–9, 190, 206, 207–8,
  234
pleasure 27, 37, 56, 63, 64, 220–1
polarity breath 215
postures (see *asana*)
power 14, 62, 148
pramada (*see* negligence)
prana 1–3, 6, 8, 11, 17, 39, 45,
  55, 79, 82, 83, 114, 120, 136,
  143, 147, 153, 154, 157, 158,
  160, 169–70, 171–3, 176,
  177, 183, 184, 187, 189–90,
  199, 200, 207, 208, 210,
  215–17, 246, 249, 251, 260
pranamaya kosha (vital sheath) 3–4,
  5, 14
prana mudra 182–3
prana vayu 4, 176
pranayama 10, 12, 24, 27, 44, 55,
  81, 112, 114, 117, 135, 138,
  142, 145, 146, 147, 150, 154,
  157, 158, 164, 169–71, 173,
  177–9, 186, 218, 219, 229,
  230, 233, 257, 260 (*see also*
  individual *pranyamas*)
pranic bath (*see* polarity breath)
pranic healing 216–17
pratyahara 24, 82, 112, 168, 200,
  213, 218–19, 223–4, 228, 233,
  257 (*see also* individual
  pratyahara techniques)
prayer 55–6, 74, 76, 153, 260–1
procrastination 72
prithvi (*see* earth)
purak (*see* inhalation)
purification 54, 115–16, 145,
  152–3 (*see also* individual
  purification techniques)
rajasic state 174

Raja Yoga 23, 111, 114, 270
ram 193
Rama, Swami 186
rechak (*see* exhalation)
rectum 160
rectus abdomini 138, 141–2
relaxation 224–5, 230, 233, 254
reproductive glands 158, 160,
  180

sabija samadhi (see *samprajnata
  samadhi*)
sabikalpa samadhi (see *samprajnata
  samadhi*)
sadhana 12
sahasrara chakra 3, 12, 13, 17, 18,
  19, 115, 155, 164, 176, 183,
  205, 251
Sai Baba, Sathya 242
salt 52, 54, 137
samadhi (superconsciousness) 13,
  18, 29, 80, 89, 111, 112, 218,
  230, 234, 244, 269–73
samana vayu 4, 176
samprajnata samadhi 270–72
samshaya (*see* doubt)
samskaras 6, 13, 96, 220, 229, 272
sananda samadhi 271
santosha (contentment) 24, 50,
  57–62, 65, 67
Saraswati, Swami Satyananda 249
sarvangasana 39–40, 226
sasmita samadhi 271
sat-chit-ananda 240
satsang 56
sattvic state 64, 75, 174, 271
satya 24, 25, 30–2
saucha 24, 50–7, 67
savichara samadhi 271
savitarka samadhi 271
savitre pranayama 214
savitri pranayama 213–14, 215,
  216, 226
Shackleton, Basil 149

security 46–7
self (see soul)
Self 7, 28, 175
self-awareness 25–6, 28, 34, 67, 69, 70, 75, 89, 91, 271
self-inquiry 27, 37, 253
self-observation 31, 32
self-realization 18, 23, 28, 30, 34, 65, 69, 76, 93, 107, 176, 232
self-study (see svadhaya)
senses 45, 61, 63, 67, 68, 69, 75, 90, 94, 148, 219–23, 228, 240–1
sensuality 14, 36
service 34, 63, 65, 76, 95, 104, 113
sexual energy 38–9, 43, 164
sexuality 13–14, 35–7, 38–9
sexual organs 159, 163
sexual problems 139
shakti (see energy)
shambhavi mudra 212
shankhaprakshalana 117, 124–35, 178
shashankasana 40, 41
shatkarmas 114, 116–17, 189 (see also individual shatkarmas)
shat kriyas 54, 112
shavasana 40, 124, 131, 132, 134, 178, 215, 216, 225, 226, 254
sheaths (see koshas)
sheetkrama kapalabhati 143
shiva (see consciousness)
Shiva 17, 84, 102, 112
Shiva Samhita 10, 112
shrine 242–3
shunya mudra 201, 202
siddhasana 39, 144, 155, 157, 158, 162, 168, 178, 193, 205, 207, 212, 246, 248–9
siddha yoni asana 157, 158, 161, 249–50
silence 31–2, 61

sinusitis 136
sirshasana 40–1
sitali pranayama 210–11
sitkari pranayama 211
Sivananda of Rishikesh, Swami 241, 244
skin 150–1, 214
sleep 6–7, 223–4
smoking 52, 57, 75, 220
soham 81, 83, 235
soul (self) 1, 6–8, 11, 17, 28, 50–1, 63, 67, 71, 87, 90–1, 94, 100, 147, 219, 221–3, 232, 234, 240, 271
sound vibration (see nada)
speech 64
sphincter muscles 158
spices 52, 54
spine 130, 131, 162, 179, 227, 259, 260
spiritual eye (ajna chakra) 10, 11, 16–18, 19, 20, 22, 29, 44, 80, 81, 82, 83, 143, 160, 161, 168, 183, 189, 193, 205, 216, 234, 235, 236, 237, 238, 260, 261, 262
spleen 119, 130, 139, 164, 260
Srimad Bhagavatam 101
stanya (see mental laziness)
stealing 33–4
stomach 119, 139
subconscious (chitta) 28–9, 173, 174, 223, 224, 225, 254
subtle pathways (see nadis)
sugar 52, 54
sukha pranayama 202–3
sukha purvaka pranayama 203
sukhasana 246, 247
sun 17, 111, 188
superconsciousness (see samadhi)
supreme Reality 59, 81, 83
survival instincts 13
surya bhedana 179
surya bedha pranayama 207

sushumna nadi 3, 11, 12, 18, 39, 83, 114, 136, 154, 156, 165, 177, 183, 187–9, 190, 204, 205, 243, 244, 260
sushupti (dreamless sleep) 1, 5
sutra neti 117, 138–9, 178
svadhaya (self-study) 50, 65–87
Svatmarama, Yogi 111, 139, 171, 172, 173
swadisthana chakra 10, 13, 22, 163
swapna (dream state) 1, 5, 224
Swara Yoga 184–9
swastikasana 178, 248

tadasana 126–7
tamasic state 64, 75, 174
Tantric Yoga 10
tapas (austerity) 50, 62–7
tea 52, 54
teeth 121–2
tejas (*see* fire)
tham 193
Teresa, Mother 93
thought 90
throat 122
thyroid glands 164, 227
tiryaka bhujangasana 128
tiryaka tadasana 128
tongue 120, 150, 165–8
tonsillitis 136
Trailanga, Swami 193
tratak 112, 117, 144–5, 236
Trinity 84
truth 30, 31, 32, 48, 60, 94–5

udana vayu 3, 176
udarakarshanasana 128
uddiyana bandha 43, 140–41, 156–7, 158, 179, 206
ujjayi pranayama 81, 83, 164, 167, 209–10
unconscious mind 32, 224, 225
upper breathing (*see* clavicular breathing)

urinary problems 123, 125, 139
ustrasana 179, 180
uterus 160, 259

vagus nerves 200
vajrasana 137, 154, 162, 178, 181, 195, 201, 202, 206, 215, 246
vajroli mudra 43, 163
vamana dhauti (see *kunjal kriya*)
vama nauli 124, 142
varisara dhauti (see *ankhaprakshalana*)
vasti 112, 117, 123–4
vastra dhauti 119
vatakrama kapalabhati 143
vayus 3, 176–7, 184, 203 (*see also* individual *vayus*)
vegetarianism 53–4, 122, 134, 147, 152–4
vibhaga pranayama 201–2
vichara 270, 271
vijnanamaya kosha 5
viloma pranayama 179, 203
viparita karani mudra 44, 163, 178, 258
virasana 44
viryastambhanasana 42
Vishnu 84, 102
vishnu mudra 190, 206
Vishnu-Purana 272
vishuddhi chakra 10, 16, 21, 164, 183
visualization 225
vital sheath (see *pranamaya kosha*)
vitarka 270, 271
Vivekananda, Swami 232, 241
vrittis 60–1, 173–6, 240
vyadhi (*see* disease)
vyana vayu 3, 177
vyutkrama kapalabhati 143

waking (see *jagrat*)
water 3, 9, 10, 14, 92, 219

water purification 118–19
will 33, 34, 48, 61, 73, 108, 109, 230
will-power 18, 62, 73, 145, 148, 189
wind 117
wind purification 117–18
Word 83–4, 85, 97

yam 193
yama 24–6, 66, 218 (*see also* individual *yamas*)
yoga mudra 161–2, 200

Yogananda, Paramhansa 11, 17, 27, 56, 58, 73, 75, 76, 77, 81, 84, 93, 95–6, 98, 101, 106, 107, 109, 165, 171, 186, 222, 238, 241, 244, 250, 258, 263, 264, 265, 266, 267, 272–3
yoga nidra 224–6, 254
yogic breathing 181, 184, 194, 195–9, 201
yogic diet 152–4
yoni mudra 168, 200, 226
Yukteswar, Sri 16, 96, 250, 263, 264, 265